Stress Reduction for Lymphedema

Disclaimer and Terms of Use: No information contained in this book should be considered as medical advice. Your reliance upon information and content obtained by you at or through this publication is solely at your own risk. Solace Massage and Mindfulness or the author assumes no liability or responsibility for damage or injury to you, other persons, or property arising from any use of any product, information, idea, or instruction contained in the content or services provided to you through this book. Reliance upon information contained in this material is solely at the reader's own risk. The author has no financial interest in and receives no compensation from manufacturers of products or websites mentioned in this book.

The National Institutes of Health states that "mind and body practices generally have good safety records when done properly by a trained professional or taught by a well-qualified instructor. However, just because a practice is safe for most people doesn't necessarily mean it's safe for you. Your medical conditions or other special circumstances (such as pregnancy) may affect the safety of a mind and body practice. When considering mind and body practices, ask about the training and experience of the practitioner or teacher, and talk with that person about your individual needs. Also, don't use a mind and body practice to postpone seeing a health care provider about a health problem" (Mind and Body Practices, 2017).

ISBN-13: 978-1-7328066-8-9

ISBN: 1-7328066-8-3 (ISBN10)

Important Notes:

The tips discussed in this book were compiled through reviewing research studies and published literature on mindfulness, interviewing experts, and listening to clients. Experts may disagree and scientific advances may render some of this information outdated. The author assumes no responsibility for any outcome of applying the information in this book for self-care. If you have any safety-related questions about the application of techniques discussed in this book, please consult your physician or mental health provider.

For Cam

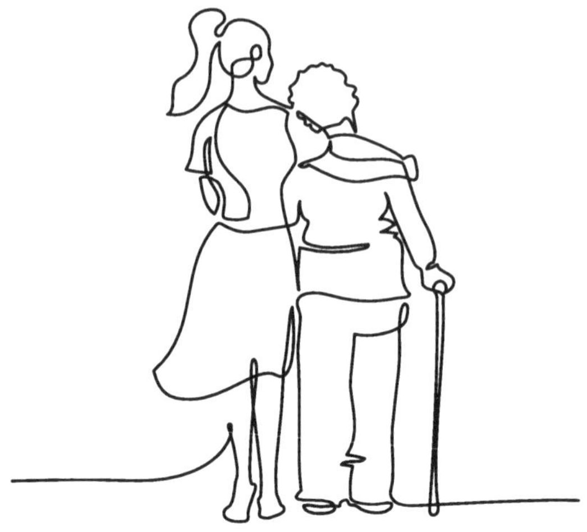

LETTER TO LYMPHEDEMA THERAPISTS

"Diminished quality of life is a complication for breast cancer survivors living with lymphedema." (Dominick et al., 2014)

A Note for Lymphedema Therapists: Why Recommend this book to your patients?

"One more thing."

If you are like most clinicians, you are wary of adding one more thing to an already packed schedule. We are busy, and our clients are often overwhelmed, juggling work and family obligations with the constant chore of managing a chronic illness. Sure, stress reduction is a nice goal, but how can we look our clients in the eye and convince them to give up 10–20 more minutes of their day for self-care?

The first thing to know is that many, many of our clients are open to learning more about complementary medicine. Australian researchers found that half of survey respondents reported using complementary and alternative medicine (CAM) therapies to treat their lymphedema (Finnane et al., 2011).

There is no one-size-fits-all prescription for stress reduction, so I have filled this book with choices for our clients. If they just can't imagine sitting still in meditation, perhaps walking a local labyrinth or another mind/body movement practice would work better. If they are having difficulty getting around, perhaps listening to music or practicing breathwork would be the better option.

Why is it important to get stress under control? Feeling stressed can get in the way of self-care. The wound care experts at WoundSource got it right when they stated that clients dealing with pain or feeling anxious or depressed may be more likely to skip several wound care appointments (Involving patients in care, 2022).

Four more reasons to share stress reduction techniques with your patients:

- Empowerment can lead to self-efficacy
- The nervous system can affect the lymphatic system

- Lymphedema reduces quality of life
- They may already be using complementary and alternative medicine

Let's look at each one in depth.

First, it's important to understand that empowering our patients to be involved in choosing and implementing their own positive health behaviors can really pay off. If a patient does not feel hopeful and in control of their health, they may not follow their treatment plan. Our wound care colleagues have seen that this is true. Patients who are actively involved in their own healthcare are more motivated to care for their own health and wellness (Involving patients in care, 2022). As clinicians, we can help clients with lymphedema diagnoses become actively involved and provide them with resources to better understand their chronic illness.

Second, stress can have an effect on our body's lymphatic system, because the nervous and lymphatic systems are interlinked. Specifically, the body's sympathetic nervous system innervates the peripheral lymphatic system (Le & Sloan, 2016) as well as secondary lymphoid organs and the larger lymphatic system in the gut (Singh et al., 2014). According to scientists at the University of Iowa in the United States of America (USA), the sympathetic nervous system expresses the fight-or-flight response, which is pro-inflammatory, and the parasympathetic system has an anti-inflammatory effect on the organs and the entire body (Singh et al.,

2014). How can this affect our body's lymphatic system? Scientists in Australia have demonstrated that chronic stress can change lymphatic vessels and cause tumor cells to spread faster (Le & Sloan, 2016).

Third, lymphedema reduces quality of life. Health-related quality of life measurements capture how a person's physical, mental and social functioning are impacted by their state of health/illness. Researchers from the UK conducted a review of the literature and found that health-related quality of life is reduced in people with lymphedema. Are we addressing this impact? If their limb is smaller and they say they are able to cope with their lymphedema, should we pat ourselves on the back and send them on their way? Are we using the right criteria to evaluate lymphedema management if we focus more on the tape measure than quality of life in people with lymphedema?

Research has found that:

- "increased limb volume is poorly related to the impact of lymphoedema on the patient"; and
- "while the women in this study appeared to cope well on a day-to-day basis, lymphoedema and its related problems were capable of inducing considerable levels of stress"

(Morgan et al., 2005).

Finally, it's important to know that our clients may already be using similar treatments and would welcome evidence-based information on stress reduction. Australian researchers sent a survey to 247 members of the Lymphedema Association of Queensland and found that, in addition to using mainstream medicine treatments for lymphedema, half of the respondents reported using at least one of 22 complementary and alternative medicine (CAM) therapies to treat their lymphedema. CAM therapies included acupuncture, aromatherapy, meditation, tai chi and yoga (Finnane et al., 2011).

Let's look at more expert opinions on sharing stress relief practices as a part of caring for clients with lymphedema.

Terence Ryan from University of Oxford states that "in the management of the swollen leg, the nature of care deserves a rethink of how best practice can relieve pain and anxiety by the release of endorphins or by switching the autonomic nervous system towards the vagal from the sympathetic" (Ryan, 2019).

Ryan is not alone in this recommendation. The call to address stress reduction is showing up more and more in the literature. Anderson and Armer conducted a literature review to identify successful intervention strategies for Breast Cancer Related Lymphedema (BCRL) among Latina survivors and state that "breast cancer survivors, in general, and survivors experiencing BCRL, specifically, have been shown to benefit from physical activity, healthy eating, lower BMI, and lower stress levels" (2021).

Shani and Walter conducted an integrative review and state that African-American cancer survivors across demographic backgrounds "have expressed receptiveness to interventions incorporating mindfulness, meditation, yoga, tai chi, and other mind-body or complementary/alternative medicine interventions" and view them as an "acceptable way to improve quality of life, pain interference, fatigue, anxiety, depression, and physical health; however, the interventions should be culturally appropriate and accessible" (2022).

The call to include stress reduction in lymphedema care is being heard at patient-focused events as well. The 2019 Lymphatic Education & Research Network's Lymphedema Patient Symposium featured a presentation titled "Addressing the Emotional Stress of Living with a Chronic Disease" delivered by Oncology Social Worker Leora Lowenthal. Lowenthal states "suffering to me is more than just physical pain.... I watch people suffer and I wonder if maybe there's more that can be done" (Lymphatic Education & Research Network, 2019).

Many of us have a lot of experience in encouraging our clients to eat well and keep active. We may have less experience in starting conversations around stress reduction. Sharing the practices found in this book is a good start.

- Kathleen Helen Lisson, CLT

"Lymphedema may cause or exacerbate emotional distress, and those with greater lymphedema-related distress have been found to have worse physical and mental health outcomes." (Gandhi et al., 2023)

FORWARD

Who doesn't feel some level of stress these days? In a fast-paced and often overwhelming world filled with competing demands for our attention, stress has become an inevitable part of our daily lives. We may constantly find ourselves racing against time, juggling multiple responsibilities, and trying to meet the ever-growing expectations of ourselves and others. As part of maintaining our own mental health and wellness, no one would disagree that it is crucial for us to find effective ways to reduce its impact and seek solace in self-care.

If you're reading this book, you may have already encountered one of the most challenging and often misunderstood diseases affected by stress – lymphedema. Often occurring as a side effect of cancer treatment, lymphedema is a chronic and progressive disease that causes the accumulation of lymph fluid in certain parts of the body, leading to discomfort, swelling, and restricted mobility. Not to mention the psychosocial effects of looking or feeling different in everyday situations and settings.

Living with a rare disease might feel like you are steering a ship at sea with no map, no friends, and no way to find your way back home. In short, I never met anyone who faked lymphedema but have met many who have faked being okay while feeling completely and utterly lost. Combating this chronic illness becomes even more critical as it compounds the burden of stress already weighing on our shoulders.

Make no mistake. Lymphedema is not just a little swelling. It can be a complete physical, emotional, and mental toll on the mind and body. It can also be an incredible financial burden and time-consuming. How do I know? I developed 3rd generation Lymphedema Distichiasis Syndrome, a rare type of primary lymphedema that affects my legs and eyes in 1994, which means my entire adult life. It has run in my family for over a century and 6 family members have been impacted with lower extremity lymphedema in various presentations.

Years ago, in 2015 I cofounded a platform with my father, Pete, called Lymphie Strong with one mission; to empower individuals with lymphedema via an online global patient support community. Sharing my family's own experiences, we hoped to inspire others to find a journey of strength and resilience. My father endured over 100 bouts of cellulitis in his lifetime and fought sepsis 3 times, so we understood the challenges and frustrations of living with lymphedema and strived to provide a safe and nurturing space for individuals to connect, learn, and advocate for lymphatic disorders of all types.

Later Lymphie Strong launched the Move That Lymph exercise series to incorporate the movement aspect of lymphatic self-care. It was during this time that I first met Kathleen Lisson online in 2017 as a member of the Lymphie Strong community. A year later, we met in person at the 3rd Annual LE&RN Run/Walk to Fight Lymphatic Disease in Santa Monica, CA where we walked the entire 5K trail together on the beach. It was serendipitous, and I am so honored to have grown in my own personal lymphedema journey with her since then.

With a passion for helping others, Kathleen has dedicated her career to providing support, education, and treatment options to individuals living with lymphedema. She understands where patients may have been failed in the past and goes above and beyond to ensure that they are armed with the latest research and information. In addition to her therapy practice, Kathleen Lisson is a prominent figure in the lymphatic world and a published author, sharing her insights and expertise in books such as "Lipedema Treatment Guide" and "Swollen, Bloated and Puffy" These resources provide valuable information on self-care, exercise, nutrition, and other lifestyle factors that can positively impact lymphedema management.

"Stress Reduction for Lymphedema" serves as a guiding light amidst the darkness. It aims to provide you with new insights, practical techniques, and empowering advice to not only tame stress but also find ways to alleviate the symptoms of lymphedema. It also shines a light on the much-needed area of mental health for lymphedema patients along with other opportunities for improvement. Throughout these pages, you will embark on a journey of self-discovery, gaining a deeper understanding of how stress influences lymphedema and ways you can cope that might not have otherwise considered and that do not necessarily cost anything. Most importantly, it is backed by empirical evidence and research.

Thank you, my dear friend Kathleen, for your ever forward-thinking vision, your innovative book, and for your tenacious spirit to make the lymphatic world better for all globally.

Veronica Poncio Seneriz

TABLE OF CONTENTS

INTRODUCTION

Thanks so much for picking up this book about stress reduction for lymphedema. I am a lymphedema therapist, and I wrote this book to provide my clients with the tools they need to reduce their stress levels.

We'll start by looking at the impact that lymphedema has on the body and mind. Then we'll take a look at stress and why stress reduction is important for our health. After that, we'll get to the fun part—learning about the different ways to reduce stress, including research on how different practices affect people with lymphedema. We'll look at:

- Working with the Breath
- Working with the Mind
- Working with the Body
- Working with Movement
- Working with the Senses
- Working with Community

I was struck by this quote from an article published in the European Journal of Oncology Nursing:

"Many patients prioritise reducing the symptom burden, increasing function, and improving quality of life over changes in swelling" (Valois et al., 2012).

I heard the message loud and clear—lymphedema therapists need to focus on more than just treatments that can reduce swelling. I was surprised at the amount of research I found on the effects of mind-body practices that focused on people with lymphedema. Where I couldn't find research on people with lymphedema, I looked for research involving people in cancer treatment. I am pleased to be able to include research involving participants with primary and secondary lymphedema, upper and lower limb lymphedema, lymphatic filariasis and podoconiosis. I hope this book informs and inspires you to take steps to reduce your stress levels. Let's get started!

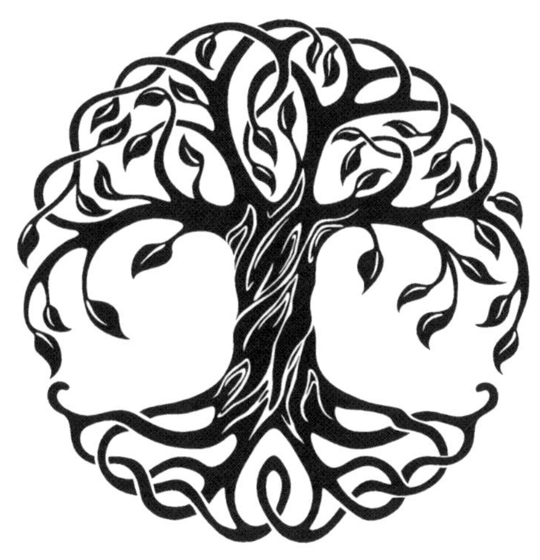

CHAPTER 1

LYMPHEDEMA AND STRESS: WHAT HAPPENS TO THE BODY?

The overly simple explanation of secondary lymphedema is that something happened to the body's lymphatic system and resulting backup of fluid in the body is causing damage and swelling.

Unfortunately, lymphedema isn't just a 'too much fluid in the wrong place' problem. Researchers from Texas A&M and Vanderbilt University in the USA share that the effects of lymphedema start before limb swelling can be noticed by others. First, the body's interstitial fluid and macromolecular proteins that are usually taken away by the lymphatic system will begin to accumulate in the tissues. This will then cause sustained inflammation, which results in tissue fibrosis and the expansion of subcutaneous adipose tissue in the immediate area (Duhon et al., 2022).

The OTHER Kind of Stress - Oxidative Stress

Most of this book is going to focus on our nervous system response to stressful situations. But first, let's look at an internal type of stress—oxidative stress. What is oxidative stress? We often think of stress as an out-of-control situation occurring outside of the body, but the body can have stress when its internal environment is out of balance as well. Oxidative stress occurs when there is an imbalance between the production of reactive oxygen species (ROS), also known as free radicals, and the body's antioxidant defenses. The vast majority of ROS are produced by our body's mitochondria (remember the electron transport chain from high school biology?) and ROS needs to be handled by the body's antioxidant enzyme systems. An imbalance in ROS is a factor in several chronic diseases, and German researchers found that ROS can also disturb lymphatic contractions (Siems et al., 2002).

Why is this important for people with lymphedema? German researchers studied the effects of manual lymphatic drainage (MLD) on people with secondary lymphedema by taking blood samples before and after MLD and again after compression was applied, and found differences between cancer survivors with lymphedema and without. The researchers described "interrelationships between oxidative stress and fibrogenesis" and recommend that reducing ROS formation and "strengthening of antioxidative defense mechanisms" should be a part of treating chronic lymphedema. In fact, the authors stated that "one can conclude that the higher the volume of the lymphoedema fluid, the higher the oxidative stress for the whole organism" (Siems et al., 2002).

How can people with lymphedema help their body reduce oxidative stress?

Research has found that lymphedematous tissue can cause excessive oxidative stress with an increase in oxidative stress levels seen when lymphedema fluid volume increases. Taiwanese researchers performed LVA supermicrosurgery on 26 people with long standing unilateral lower limb lymphedema. Patients wore custom-made compression stockings after surgery. The researchers found "reductions in some specific oxidative stress markers and improved antioxidant capacity" after the surgical intervention (Yang et al., 2021).

What are some nonsurgical ways to affect oxidative stress?

Deep breathing may help reduce oxidative stress. Italian researchers had athletes practice deep breathing after a hard training session and found that "relaxation induced by diaphragmatic breathing increases the antioxidant defense status in athletes after exhaustive exercise. These effects correlate with the concomitant decrease in cortisol and the increase in melatonin. The consequence is a lower level of oxidative stress, which suggests that an appropriate diaphragmatic breathing could protect athletes from long-term adverse effects of free radicals" (Martarelli et al, 2011). We will learn more about diaphragmatic breathing later in the book.

In the article "Strategies for reducing or preventing the generation of oxidative stress," Borut Poljsak from the University of Ljubljana's Laboratory for Oxidative Stress Research in Slovenia recommends regular moderate exercise, quality sleep, taking time for relaxation and hobbies, and avoiding excessive psychophysical stress (Poljsak, 2011). But wait, shouldn't we try to eliminate all stress from our life and pop antioxidant supplements to reduce oxidative stress? A better way may be to trigger the body's adaptive stress response through moderate exercise and positive stress. The result? Our system will activate our endogenous, or internal, antioxidant and damage-repair processes.

Now, let's learn more about psychological and physical stress.

Psychosocial Impact of Lymphedema

"Healthcare professionals who deal with patients who have venous disease, lymphatic malformations, or secondary lymphedema are uniquely positioned to help address psycho-social issues in these patients." (Sheila Ridner, Vanderbilt University)

When lymphedema gets worse, it's not just the tissue that is affected. Brazilian researchers studying women with Breast Cancer Related Lymphedema (BCRL) found that chronic lymphedema caused both physical effects in the tissue of the affected arm and psychological stress, and that both worsen as the lymphedema progresses (Perez et al., 2022). USA researchers conducted a San Diego, California-based study that found over 48% of women with BCRL who answered the question "How much does your lymphedema distress or bother you?" indicated moderate to extreme distress (Dominick et al., 2014).

The negative effects of stressors start even before the cancer survivor is diagnosed with lymphedema. Spanish researchers looking at the effects of health interventions on people with breast cancer found that about thirty percent of those with breast cancer have an anxiety disorder more than 5 years after diagnosis, which may result in an increased stress hormone response. Fear plays a big part. The researchers recommend therapies that "reduce negative feelings related to the fear of disease progression and the risk of recidivism and that promote positive emotions and better coping" (Obrero-Gaitán et al., 2022).

Fear is a stressor that has a huge impact on our lives. What other issues are causing stress? Some of the top themes that cause psychosocial stress for people with lymphedema involve not getting their needs met. These include:

- Lack of lymphedema research
- Lack of treatment resources
- Lack of insurance coverage for treatment and supplies
- Healthcare professionals who don't communicate an understanding of the seriousness of the patient's problems
- Parental despair when lymphedema happens to a child

(Ridner, 2009).

Canadian researchers interviewed people with lower limb lymphedema and found that they experienced isolation and uncertainty (Bowman et al., 2021). Researchers in Nepal interviewed people with lymphatic filariasis and found that they experience stress, anxiety, low self-esteem, worry, and fear of abandonment. Some women reported fear of transmitting the disease to children (Adhikari et al., 2015).

How does lymphedema change the experience of living in one's own body? Cancer-related lymphedema brings or intensifies additional burdens over and above those experienced as a result of the cancer diagnosis and treatment. Women with lymphedema have different symptoms from those without lymphedema, including psychological distress, fatigue, decreased physical activity, loss of confidence in their body, and altered limb sensation (Ridner, 2009).

Expressive writing is one way to cope with the stressors that come with lymphedema. We can learn about the lived experience of having lymphedema from the expressive writing of people with the disease. The expressive writing of people with BCRL highlights their struggles with many of the issues listed above, as well as feelings of anger and guilt, concerns about abandonment, and embarrassment about their appearance when they are out in public (Ridner, 2009). We will learn more about expressive writing later in the book.

The psychosocial impact of lymphedema is defined as "the combination of the psychological and social factors/concerns that directly affect an individual with lymphedema." (Fu et al., 2012)

Let's talk about emotional frustration. What causes frustration in people with lymphedema? Researchers found that the top causes of frustration include:

- Time consuming nature of self-care

- Inability to find properly fitting clothes
- Lack of a cure
- Disinterested healthcare providers
- Lack of financial help from insurance companies
- Government and social marginalization

(Fu et al., 2012)

The bottom line is that people with lymphedema don't feel supported. Nobody has extra time in their busy schedules, yet people with lymphedema are expected to have the time and finances to participate in daily self-care. Add to this the fact that, by and large, people with lymphedema are not fully supported by the fashion industry, the medical profession, insurance companies, their government, or society.

It's important to note that the experiences of people with primary lymphedema are not exactly the same as those with secondary lymphedema. Persons with primary lymphedema have many of the same psychosocial stress issues as those with secondary lymphedema, including self-image and finding clothing that fits, and they may have greater difficulty with diagnosis and receiving treatment in a timely manner. Many of the stories of those with primary lymphedema have elements in common. Researchers spoke with people with primary lymphedema and found three common themes in their experiences: "each participant reached a point in his or her life with lymphedema when they felt they had Nowhere to Turn. Correct diagnosis and referral for inpatient care was a Turning Point for them in terms of managing lymphedema, and all were now Making Room in their lives for the complex self-management routines needing to be followed" (Bogan et al., 2007).

> *"People affected by lymphoedema often experience rejection, stigma, and discrimination. . . . However, the management of this condition has focused on prevention and treatment through drug administration, with scant attention paid to its real-life impact." (Río-González et al., 2021)*

What Happens to the Body During Stress?

Our body often reacts to stressful situations by activating the "fight-or-flight" sympathetic nervous system so we are ready to respond to threats. In the short term, raising our heart rate and reducing our digestion can help us focus our energy on escaping an alligator attack (for instance), but chronic activation of the sympathetic nervous system can result in constant production of hormones like cortisol, which increases glucose in the bloodstream and suppresses digestion, and catecholamines, which increase blood pressure and reduce blood flow to the skin.

The stressful situation can also come from our thoughts. Germer and Neff state that "self-criticism activates the threat defense system... When we feel in danger, the amygdala sends signals that increase blood pressure, adrenaline and the hormone cortisol" (Germer & Neff, 2019).

We have all heard about the negative effects of stressors on our health. Is there any special concern for people with lymphedema? Lymphedema often results in impaired immune function (Yuan et al., 2019) and skin changes. The health of our skin is important because it is one of our first lines of defense. Impaired immune function and a weakened skin barrier can leave the body vulnerable to infection. Researchers from the USA state that "more than 300 studies have shown that psychological stress is capable of a dose-related modification of the immune system. Behavior and stress are postulated to enter the body through sympathetic fibers descending from the brain into bone marrow, thymus, spleen, and lymph nodes" (McClure et al., 2010) and USA and Canadian researchers state that "these fibers can release a wide variety of substances that influence immune responses by binding to receptors on white blood cells" (Segerstrom & Miller, 2004).

What happens to the body as a result of exposure to ongoing stressful situations? Romanian researchers explain that "enduring stress, which is known to result in down-regulation of beta-adrenergic receptors, alters adhesion molecules expression on leukocytes, with a resultant decrease of immune response to acute psychological challenges in chronically stressed persons. In contrast to acute stress, chronic stress impairs NK and T cell function" (Dragos & Tănăsescu, 2010). Chronic stress weakens our immune response, a situation which is even more dangerous in those with lymphedema.

Lymphedema affects the skin. This is why skin care is taught as a part of complex decongestive therapy. Why is skin health so important? The Romanian researchers explain that intact, healthy skin serves as a barrier to prevent the entry of pathogens. When a person experiences short- or long-term psychological stress, wounds may heal slower and injured skin may take longer to heal. The researchers explain that "the slow resolution of skin injuries is attributed to stress-induced neural, endocrine and immune alterations: activation of immune and inflammatory processes in the skin, neuropeptide release from the peripheral nerves, and increased systemic glucocorticoid levels. These neural, endocrine and immune changes interfere with processes such as lipid synthesis and cytokine expression, important in the initial phases of wound healing" (Dragos & Tănăsescu, 2010).

Conclusion

We have learned that lymphedema is much more than too much fluid. Inflammation plays a role as well. Lifestyle choices and chronic lymphedema can result in oxidative stress, which has been linked to fibrogenesis and the increased production of Reactive Oxygen Species, which can disturb lymphatic contractions (Siems et al., 2002). Lymphedema symptoms often result in psychosocial stress in people with the disease, whether they have primary or secondary lymphedema. We wrapped up this chapter by looking at the negative effects of acute and chronic stress for people with lymphedema, including effects on the immune system and skin health.

Though this book will focus on stress reduction practices for lymphedema, it is critical to understand that lymphedema management must be at the top of our self-care list. No amount of breathing exercises and expressive writing can overcome the negative effects of unmanaged lymphedema. Researchers from the USA found that “lymphedema progresses in intensity and grade without adherence to treatment” (McClure et al., 2010). This applies not just to secondary lymphedema after cancer, but to all types of lymphedema. Ethiopian researchers took a look at the experiences of people with podoconiosis, a disease impacting the lower extremity lymph vessels caused by exposure to irritants in soil, and state that “lymphedema management is effective in improving clinical outcomes and the quality of life of people affected with podoconiosis” (Abebaw et al., 2022). Treat lymphedema first, then address stress reduction.

Now let’s look at how we can measure stress levels in the body and some practices that can help reduce the effects of stressors. We will start with practices that work with the breath, then explore practices that work with the mind, then the body. and finish with practices that work with the community.

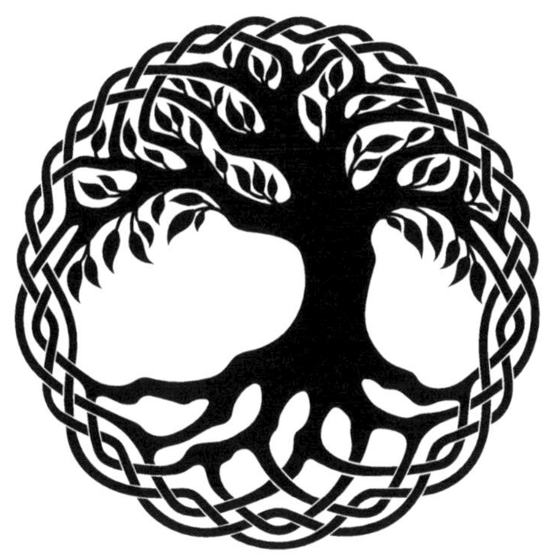

CHAPTER 2
STRESS REDUCTION PRACTICES

What do we mean when we talk about stress reduction? There are two ways to reduce the burden of stressors on our bodies. We can reduce the number of stressful situations and we can increase our capacity to handle those stressful situations. Most of us cannot easily change jobs and reduce our responsibilities to family and community, so we'll focus on increasing our capacity to handle those stressful situations by looking at opportunities to activate our body's relaxation response.

Relaxation Response

What is the relaxation response? The term was first described by Herbert Benson, founder of the Mind/Body Medical Institute at Massachusetts General Hospital in Boston. The relaxation response is the counterpart of the body's stress response. Why is the relaxation response so valuable to those of us with recurring stressors in our lives? Spending more time with our parasympathetic nervous system in charge allows it to modulate incoming fight-or-flight sympathetic activity (Rio-Alamos et al., 2023). Stress reduction practices including yoga, meditation, and repetitive prayer can create the relaxation response, which may improve mitochondrial resiliency (Balasubramanian, 2015).

Stress and Heart Rate Variability

Heart Rate Variability (HRV) is one way we can measure our body's stress levels. What is heart rate variability? Our heart and brain communicate with each other. The variation in the frequency of time between our heartbeats can be affected by interactions of our sympathetic and parasympathetic nervous system. HRV can be measured by an electrocardiogram machine (EKG). A higher HRV is a sign that we have lower stress levels and can adapt to change. A lower HRV can be a sign of health issues (Heart Rate Variability, 2021).

What does the evidence show? Researchers from the USA performed a literature review on HRV research and found evidence that HRV affects decision-making. Higher HRV is linked to:

- Emotional regulation
- Greater executive function
- Better dietary decisions
- Better control over social media use
- Better negativity avoidance

They concluded that higher HRV-based behaviors can "benefit health and wellbeing" (Arakaki et al., 2023).

Italian researchers did a scoping review of heart rate variability biofeedback in cancer patients and found that HRV is associated with:

- Cognitive resilience
- Emotional regulation
- Modulation of cortisol, cardiovascular and inflammatory responses

(Spada et al., 2022).

Stay tuned—several of the studies I will share later in the book will use HRV as a measurement.

Cortisol

Cortisol is another important measurement of our body's stress response. Researchers from Sweden and the UK state that "cortisol is a glucocorticoid hormone that plays a vital role in the physiological response to endogenous and exogenous stressors in the human body." Why is it important to be aware of cortisol levels in the body? The researchers state that "cortisol's immunosuppressive effect may result in reduced immunosurveillance of early-stage cancer, facilitating their immune escape and acquisition of further oncogenic mutations" (Larsson et al., 2021).

Relaxation Sensitivity / Relaxation Induced Anxiety

Everybody wants to relax, right? Not everybody. Relaxation Sensitivity and the resulting Relaxation Induced Anxiety (RIA) happens when someone perceives the feelings related to relaxation as negative instead of positive and soothing. **Up to 54% of people with anxiety may experience this discomfort.** They may experience relaxation as a "loss of control, increased self-focus or worrisome or disturbing thoughts." People can also feel like taking time to relax makes them appear unmotivated or lazy to others (Luberto et al., 2021). Researchers found that over 30% of people with chronic tension experienced RIA when practicing progressive muscle relaxation and over 53% of people with chronic tension experienced RIA when practicing mantra meditation (Kim & Newman, 2019). It may be useful to know that it's okay if relaxation techniques leave us feeling neutral. We did not 'fail' at relaxing if we did not feel calm, patient and restored after every practice. If you find that you are really struggling with feeling comfortable relaxing, speaking to a mental health professional may help.

> *"High levels of evidence support the routine use of mind-body practices, such as yoga, meditation, relaxation techniques and passive music therapy to address common mental health concerns among breast cancer patients, including anxiety, stress, depression, and mood disturbances. Additionally, meditation has been shown to improve quality of life and physical functioning, and yoga has been found to improve quality of life and fatigue." (Greenlee et al., 2017)*

Conclusion

We learned about the Relaxation response and heart rate variability as a way to measure stress reduction. We finished up by taking a look at Relaxation Sensitivity / Relaxation Induced Anxiety, two important concepts to understand before we practice new mindfulness techniques. Now, let's look at how to work with the breath to reduce the impact of stress in the body.

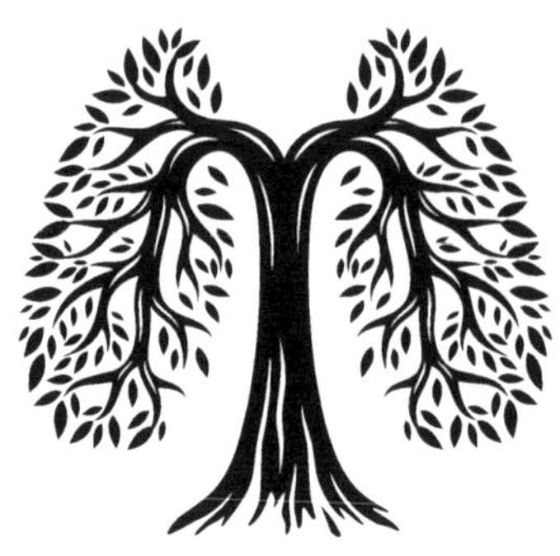

CHAPTER 3

WORKING WITH THE BREATH

Let's begin this chapter with a quick breathwork technique you can use anywhere to help you focus and reorient to the present moment.

The STOP technique was created by Jon Kabat-Zinn to get us off "autopilot." Let's try it now.

The steps are:

- Stop (stop what we are doing for a moment)
- Take a Breath (pay attention as you take the next breath)

- Observe (what are your current feelings and emotions? Are there any notable physical sensations in your body? We don't need to change or judge them, just observe them)
- Proceed (return to what we were doing before)

What to Know Before You Start

If breathwork were as easy as sitting and taking a few slow, deep breaths, I wouldn't have much to write about in this chapter. First, it's important to realize that breathwork is not an enjoyable and productive experience for everyone. I have heard people tell me many times that mindfulness "doesn't work" for them because they cannot sit still and/or they tried to pay attention to their breathing and found themselves constantly bombarded by thoughts. Having thoughts is completely normal, but they think it means they are a failure at meditating. In fact, the power of meditation is training ourselves to have equanimity when we find ourselves thinking and gently redirecting ourselves back to the breath without self-blame or anger.

People who have unrealistic personal standards, are very concerned about their mistakes, and seem focused on failure may have maladaptive perfectionism. They seem like the ideal candidate for mindfulness because too much focus on perfectionistic thinking is associated with chronic stress and rumination, and maladaptive perfectionism can get in the way of relaxation. Unfortunately, experts have found that perfectionists may not get stress-reduction benefits from mindfulness practices that just focus on the breath. Perfectionists may want to avoid unpleasant sensations and thoughts, and the experience of feeling like they cannot keep focus on the breath may cause them to experience that they are a failure at meditating (Azam et al., 2015). What can we do if we feel like we are “failing” at meditating? Those who are self-critical may benefit from trying self-compassion meditation first (Neff, n.d.). I will share information about self-compassion meditation later in the book.

It is important to be aware that people who have a trauma history may find breathwork triggering. Deep breathing may be counterproductive if we are already hyperventilating, which may happen during periods of anxiety or stress. Seek out a trauma-informed meditation teacher to serve as a resource, rather than trying to struggle through learning meditation practices without support.

Now that we have looked at what to be aware of before we try breathwork, let’s look at some breathwork practices.

Diaphragmatic Breathing

If you have had manual lymphatic drainage, chances are that your lymphedema therapist incorporated diaphragmatic breathing into your session. The diaphragm is a dome-shaped muscle located at the base of the lungs. There are several muscles the body uses to breathe, but the diaphragm is the one we encourage you to move the most during breathing. Why? Because using the diaphragm can improve lymphatic drainage in the body.

Polish researchers found that the localized lymphatic drainage system that serves the diaphragm works to absorb fluid from the body's peritoneal cavity and diverts it into the vascular system (Kocjan et al., 2017). The peritoneum is the tissue that lines your abdominal wall and covers abdominal organs. Why is this so useful? Because over half of our body's lymph nodes are underneath the diaphragm. When our diaphragm expands and contracts to facilitate breathing, those lymph nodes are also pulling lymphatic fluid through the system (Kocjan et al., 2017).

It is important to regularly breathe with our diaphragm, because moving lymphatic fluid depends on expansion and contraction of the diaphragm as well as intraperitoneal pressure and our body's posture (lying down, sitting or standing) (Kocjan et al., 2017). Diaphragmatic breathing may also feel soothing and reduce our stress levels.

Let's feel the difference between breathing more with our diaphragm and breathing using our accessory muscles of breathing. First, let's use our diaphragm and intercostal muscles (located in between our ribs) and feel them expand and contract. This first exercise is based on a breathwork technique by Carl Stough.

- Exhale fully and pull your belly button in toward your spine gently
- Take a nice deep breath, feeling your abdomen and belly button naturally move forward (you don't have to focus on moving them out)
- As you exhale, whisper the numbers from 1-10 over and over
- As you run out of air, keep on repeating them even though you can't hear yourself
- Feel how tight and close to your spine your ribcage is as you exhale
- Take a deep breath and feel your ribcage expand in all directions as you inhale

Now, let's take a breath using mostly our accessory breathing muscles like the scalenes by our neck and intercostal muscles in between our ribs.

- Exhale fully and pull your belly button in toward your spine gently and firmly
- Hold your belly button toward the spine and don't allow your belly to expand as you breathe
- Take a full breath
- Feel your lungs expanding nearer to the top of your ribcage

- Exhale
- Let the belly button relax and breathe normally

This upper chest type of breathing may feel familiar to many people. We may have trained ourselves to suck our tummy in to appear smaller or wear tight clothing that doesn't let our belly move in and out as we breathe.

Neither of these two practices is a recommended way to breathe throughout the day. They are just to let us feel the different muscles that can control breathing. Now, let's practice the type of breathing we DO recommend—what we call diaphragmatic breathing.

Diaphragmatic Breathing

- Begin in a relaxed yet alert position
- Place one hand just below your rib cage
- Breathe in slowly through your nose (or mouth if you cannot breathe through your nose) so that your abdomen moves out against your hand
- Your upper chest should remain relatively still
- Breathe out through your nose or mouth as your belly button moves in toward the spine

How do you feel during and after diaphragmatic breathing?

___

___

___

Find more information on diaphragmatic breathing here:

https://my.clevelandclinic.org/health/articles/9445-diaphragmatic-breathing

This type of breathing is also practiced during yoga asana sessions tailored for people with lymphedema. Researchers in India recommend that patients use long, diaphragmatic breaths and focus their eyes on a point in front of them, usually on the wall or floor (Narahari et al., 2016). Researchers from the Centre for Neglected Tropical Diseases recommend that people with lymphatic filariasis- and podoconiosis-related lymphedema take five deep diaphragmatic breaths on five occasions during the day as part of enhanced-care activities to support lymphatic flow (Douglass et al., 2019).

Researchers from Bangladesh and the UK found that a protocol of lymphatic stimulating activities in people affected by moderate and severe lymphedema filariasis resulted in "significant improvement in lymphedema status and reduction in acute attacks" and greater improvements were seen in the group who "performed lymphatic stimulating activities such as self-massage and deep breathing as part of their daily lymphedema self-care" when tissue compressibility was considered (Douglass et al, 2020b). The lead researcher also found similar results for people with moderate and severe lower-limb lymphedema in the Simada District in north western Ethiopia, which "has a high prevalence of LF-related lymphedema and is co-endemic for podoconiosis" (Douglass et al., 2020a).

Diaphragmatic breathing can also be beneficial for the whole family. Chinese researchers developed a protocol of "resting breathing for 15 min and diaphragmatic breathing for 15 min in each session" for healthy adults. Participants conducted 20 sessions over an 8 week period. Researchers concluded that "diaphragmatic breathing could improve sustained attention, affect, and cortisol levels" (Ma et al., 2017).

Which type of breath felt most comfortable to you? Were you surprised at how narrow your rib cage could get during the exhale in the 1-10 breathing? Did any of the breath exercises make you feel anxious? Did any make you feel calmer?

____

____

____

Cyclic Sighing

Cyclic sighing consists of taking a two-part deep inhale and a longer exhale. Practicing can bring an increase in positive affect as well as “psychological relief, shifts in autonomic states, and resetting of respiratory rate” and the effects are cumulative—benefits increase as the exercise is practiced regularly (Balban et al., 2023).

Let’s try cyclic sighing:

- Begin in a relaxed yet alert position. Your eyes can be open or closed
- Exhale fully
- Breath in through your nose
- When your lungs feel full, take another, shorter inhale through the nose to fully inflate your lungs
- Exhale slowly
- Repeat for a total of 5 minutes

Box Breathing

Box breathing, also called tactical breathing, uses equal ratios of inhalation, exhalation and breath holding and has been used by the military for “stress regulation and performance improvement” (Balban et al., 2023).

Let’s try four rounds of box breathing:

- Begin in a relaxed yet alert position. Your eyes can be open or closed

- Exhale fully
- Breath in for a count of 4
- Hold the breath for a count of 4
- Exhale for a count of 4
- Hold the breath for a count of 4
- Repeat three more times

4-7-8 Breathing

Let's try four rounds of 4,7,8 breathing:

- Begin in a relaxed yet alert position. Your eyes can be open or closed
- Exhale fully
- Breath in for a count of 4
- Hold the breath for a count of 7
- Exhale for a count of 8
- Repeat 3 more times

How do you feel after these short breathing interventions?

____

____

____

Slow Breathing

We just learned about different breathing techniques for stress reduction; now let's look at some research about how often to breathe.

Breathing at the rate of six breaths a minute equals a breathing frequency of 0.1 Hz. What's so special about 0.1 Hz? Changing our breathing pattern can change our autonomic nervous system activity. Specifically, slow breathing reduces the secretion of adrenal medulla norepinephrine and reduces sympathetic nerve excitement (Kai et al., 2021). Norepinephrine, also known as noradrenaline, is used in the fight-or-flight response of the sympathetic nervous system. Stressful situations can trigger the release of norepinephrine, so it's useful to use slow breathing to help reduce the secretion of this hormone.

The practice of using slow breathing to control the body's stress response may be familiar to you if you had biofeedback training as part of cancer treatment to reduce anxiety, insomnia, and chronic pain.

We just learned how slow breathing helps our nervous system. What effects does slow breathing have on the cardiopulmonary system? Australian researchers found that breathing six times per minute improves alveolar ventilation, increases arterial oxygen saturation and venous return and lowers blood pressure. Patients with chronic heart failure who practiced slow breathing found that it improved their exercise performance and motivation (Russo et al., 2017).

Slow Breathing Through Chanting

How can we breathe at a rate of 0.1 Hz? Researchers from Austria shared several different ways to breathe at 0.1 Hz, including "yogic breathing with a 4 second inhale and a 6 second exhale or reciting the Rosary, in which each Hail Mary prayer takes 10 seconds" (Tanzmeister et al., 2022).

That's right—if you are Catholic, you may already be practicing slow breathing! One traditional way to pray the Rosary is for the priest/leader to recite the first half of the Hail Mary, and the congregation to recite the second half aloud in unison. This method lets everyone take about 5 seconds for an inhale, and about 5 seconds for exhaling while reciting their half of the prayer.

A study published in the British Medical Journal found that the breathing frequency of people reciting the Hail Mary prayer "coincides with the subjects' spontaneous Mayer wave frequency and thus enhanced this cardiovascular oscillation by synchronising sympathetic and vagal outflow. This even resulted in rhythmic fluctuations in cerebral blood flow, which might directly influence central nervous oscillations" (Bernardi et al., 2001).

In addition to all its spiritual benefits, reciting the Rosary aloud can be a breathing exercise that reduces stress. In a journal article focusing on Latinas with BCRL, researchers found that psychological outcomes improved when Latinas had social support, used active coping strategies, and participated in faith-based practices. Latinas used church groups and prayer as emotional support. One woman said, "I pray using the Rosary and so that has comforted me much" (Buki et al., 2021).

If you are praying the Rosary by yourself, try using an audio recording (there are plenty on YouTube) so you can see if this style of slow breathing is right for you.

"Slow breathing causes the pulse harmonics of blood flow (i.e. blood pressure oscillations) to synchronise with the rhythm of the heart." (Russo et al., 2017)

The same researchers who investigated the Hail Mary prayer also found similar benefits to chanting the yoga mantra 'Om-Mani-Padme-Hum.' Chanting slowed breathing to around six breaths per minute as well as enhancing HRV and baroreflex sensitivity (Bernardi et al., 2001).

Let's try it! I chant a similar mantra in the mornings. First, find a recording of Om Mani Padme Hum on YouTube. I use this one: https://bit.ly/108OmManiPadmeHum

- Begin in a relaxed yet alert position. Your eyes can be open or closed

- Exhale fully
- Breathe in slowly through your nose (or mouth if you cannot breathe through your nose).
- Chant "Om Mani Padme Hum" along with the video two times in a comfortable tone (about five seconds)
- Breathe in slowly through the nose or mouth as the mantra repeats two more times (about five seconds)
- Repeat this pattern of chanting two verses, then inhaling for two verses for a total of around six minutes of chanting
- Tip: recordings of 108 repetitions of continuous chanting last around five and a half minutes

How do you feel after chanting?

____

____

____

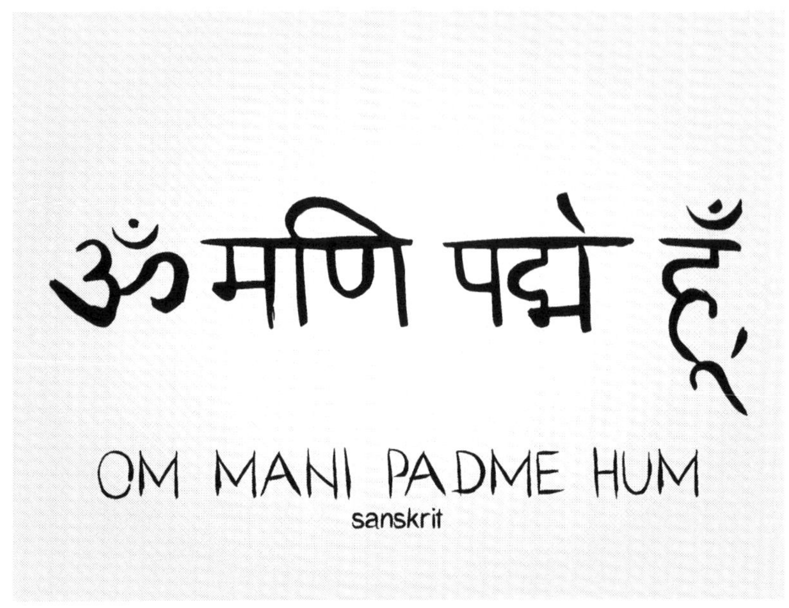

The Science Behind Singing and Chanting

Singing combines sound, vibration and the benefits of a slower breathing rate and extended exhale. Singing in a group can also enhance feelings of social connection. Researchers from the UK, including the Royal College of Music in London, took a look at the effects of singers in a choir who were in cancer treatment, cared for a loved one with a cancer diagnosis, or had lost a loved one to cancer. The study monitored the singers' mood as well as neuroendocrine, neuropeptide and immune responses. They found that an hour of choir singing resulted in an increase in positive affect and decrease in negative affect (Fancourt et al., 2016).

Researchers from Austria also found that singing under pleasant circumstances, either alone or with others, resulted in a lowered negative response to stressors, a decrease in cortisol, and increased feelings of sense of self and subjective wellbeing (Tanzmeister et al., 2022). Researchers from the USA explored the effect of religious songs on cancer-related psychological symptoms and found that "religious songs are an important strategy used among older African American cancer patients" that "might enhance health outcomes among this medically underserved cancer population" (Hamilton et al., 2016).

If you enjoy singing, whether in the shower, to a pet or loved one, or in a group, it is a good technique to lower stress.

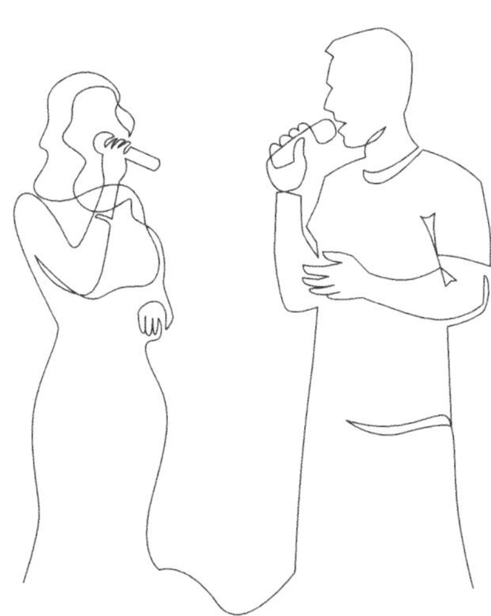

OM/AUM Chanting

Why might chanting OM/AUM reduce stress? Balasubramanian states that pranayama involves diaphragmatic breathing, which "increases vagal tone and parasympathetic dominance and decreases sympathetic discharges." He has found that, according to pilot studies, chanting OM/AUM may have the following benefits:

- Reduction of heart rate and blood pressure in hypertensive patients
- Increase in cutaneous peripheral vascular resistance
- Vagal nerve stimulation (VNS), and
- Deactivation of the limbic brain regions, amygdala, hippocampus, parahippocampal gyrus, insula, and orbitofrontal and anterior cingulate cortices and thalamus

(Balasubramanian, 2015).

Hotho et al. found that chanting the word OM/AUM may activate "neural structures involved in attention, emotions and control of the autonomic nervous system." When researchers recorded the effects of chanting OM/AUM at 0.05 Hz, which is a 20-second breath, they found that OM/AUM chanting at breathing frequencies of about three breaths per minute resulted in 0.1 Hz oscillations in systolic blood pressure (SBP) and concluded that chanting OM/AUM at this slow rate does synchronize cardiorespiratory and blood pressure oscillations (2022).

Chanting, specifically chanting the word OM/AUM, results in a slower breathing rate and increased airway resistance. The body contracts the larynx in order to produce the vibration of the different sounds in the word OM/AUM, which increases vagal tone. Increased vagal tone results in arousal of the body's parasympathetic nervous system (Anjana et al., 2022).

The technique used in the Anjana study involved chanting OM/AUM by vocalizing the O or AU sound for a third of the time and M for the other two thirds of the time. Each OM/AUM cycle took 20 seconds and the total practice took five minutes (Anjana et al., 2022).

Let's try the Anjana "Relaxation Technique" protocol:

- Begin in a relaxed yet alert position. Your eyes can be open or closed
- Exhale fully
- Breathe in slowly through your nose (or mouth if you cannot breathe through your nose)
- Sing OM/AUM in a low yet comfortable tone
- Let the O or AU last five seconds
- Let the M last 10 seconds
- Breathe in slowly through the nose or mouth
- Repeat 14 more times or until five minutes has elapsed

How do you feel after the "Relaxation Technique?"

___

___

___

Hotho didn't require participants to vocalize OM/AUM in a particular way, just to let the exhale last for 20 seconds. Instead of continuously repeating the chant, participants took a two-minute rest in between sets. Let's try the Hotho "Slow Speech Guided Breathing" protocol:

- Begin in a relaxed yet alert position. Your eyes can be open or closed
- Exhale fully
- Breathe in slowly through your nose (or mouth if you cannot breathe through your nose).
- Sing OM/AUM in a low yet comfortable tone for 20 seconds
- Breathe in slowly through the nose or mouth
- Repeat four more times
- Rest for two minutes
- Complete two more sets of five OM chants, with two minutes rest in between each set of five.

(2022)

Which way of chanting OM/AUM felt more comfortable to you?

____

____

____

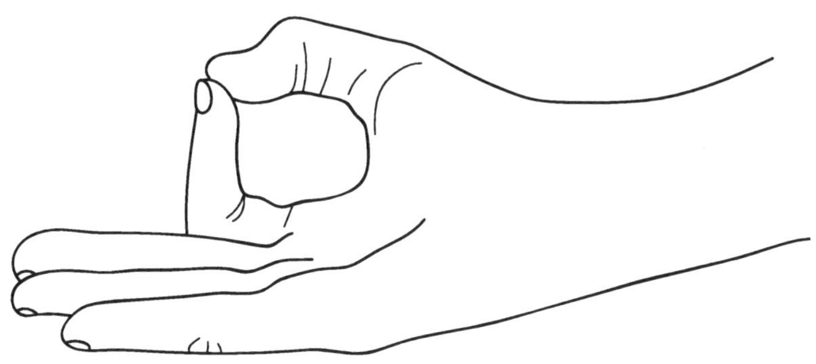

Chin Mudra

Pranayama

Pranayama practices are focused on controlling the life force in our body. Other words used to describe prana can be vitality, creative force or qi.

One of the most accessible forms of pranayama is breathwork. In *Anatomy and Physiology of Yogic Practices*, M.M. Gore states that pranayama involves practices that can enable us to control our state of mind through our breathing. Many pranayama practices specifically include pausing the breath, either after a slow inhalation or after a slow exhalation. Interestingly, after practicing pranayama for a long period of time, we may begin to notice our normal breathing speed change or our breathing pause by itself (2005).

First, let's learn about mudras. The Institute of Applied Dermatology "yoga protocol for treatment of breast cancer-related lymphedema" includes mudras with the practice of pranayama, including Chin Mudra, Mrigi Mudra and Namaskara Mudra (Narahari et al., 2016).

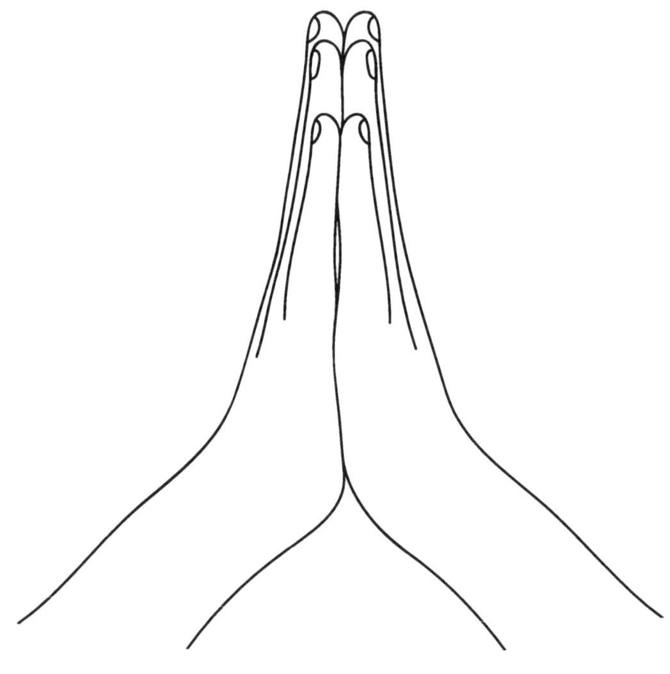

Anjali Mudra

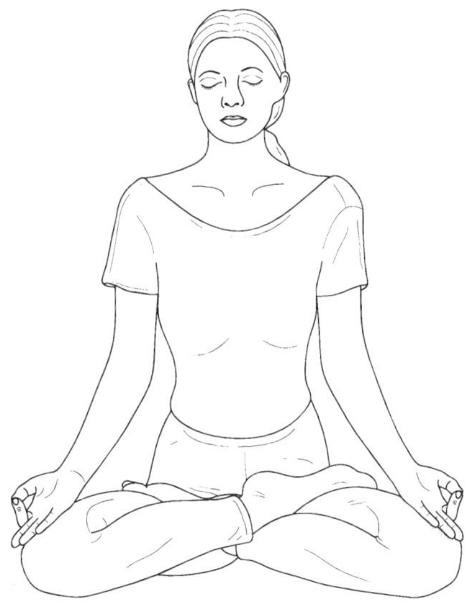

Padmasana
or Lotus Pose

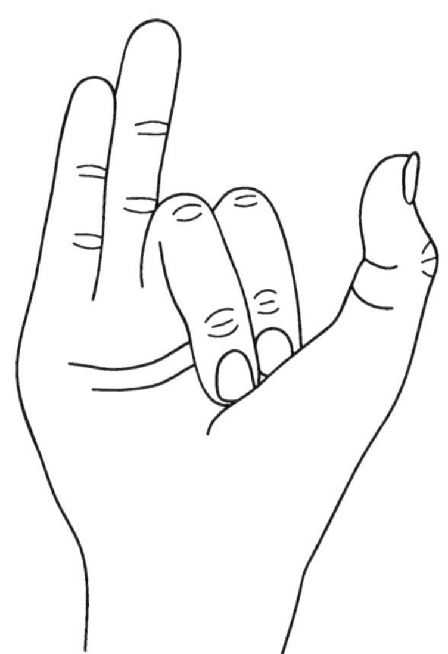

Vishnu Mudra

"Chin mudra was performed by keeping thumb and index finger flexed and joined together. Other fingers were kept straight. Both the palms were kept on the folded knee facing upward in either Padmasana or Swastikasana." (Narahari et al., 2016) Padmasana is also called Lotus pose and Swastikasana is also called Auspicious pose. "Mrigi Mudra was used to close nostrils for selective inhalation or exhalation during Pranayama. Here, the right forefinger and the middle finger were clenched while the thumb and other two fingers were kept straight." (Narahari et al., 2016) Mrigi mudra is also called Vishnu mudra. "In Namaskara Mudra, both palms and fingers were kept together touching each other." (Narahari et al., 2016) Namaskara mudra is also called Anjali mudra.

Let's investigate by trying a few short breathing exercises. We can start with left nostril breathing. We will inhale through our left nostril and exhale through our right nostril.

- Sit in a comfortable yet alert position with a straight spine
- Close your eyes, if that feels comfortable
- Take a few diaphragmatic breaths
- Use your hand held in Vishnu Mudra / Mrigi Mudra—index and middle finger held at the base of the thumb—to help you close off each nostril when needed

- Inhale slowly into the left nostril while closing the right nostril with the thumb
- Exhale with the right nostril, closing the left nostril with the ring finger
- Continue breathing this way for up to three minutes
- Release your hand and take a few deep breaths through both nostrils before ending the practice

How do you feel after left nostril breathing?

____

____

____

Indian researchers designed a study to test the effects of different types of nostril breathing on heart rate variability, skin conductance, breath rate, and blood pressure.

The protocol was:

- 5 minutes of sitting quietly
- 30 minutes of breathing practice
- 5 minutes of sitting quietly

The researchers found that a session of:

- Right nostril breathing resulted in an increase in systolic, diastolic and mean pressure

- Left nostril breathing resulted in a decrease in systolic and mean pressure
- Alternate nostril breathing resulted in a decrease in systolic and diastolic pressure

The researchers state that "right unilateral forced nostril breathing is associated with a generalized increase in sympathetic tone." The researchers note that prior research found that right nostril breathing "significantly increased blood glucose while left nostril breathing lowered it" and "left nostril yoga breathing also increased the volar galvanic skin resistance (suggestive of a decrease in sympathetic activity)" (Raghuraj & Telles, 2008).

Bhastrika

Bhastrika is a more intense and quick form of breathwork. It is best to practice this type of breathwork on an empty stomach. Try practicing in the morning before exercise or breakfast.

Narahari includes it in the treatment protocol for BCRL because of its effects on lymphatic flow. The article states that "controlled breathing along with contraction of rectus abdominis, diaphragm, and intercostal muscles as in Bhastrika creates pressure differences in both abdomen and thoracic region. These pressure differences allow lymph to drain toward the thorax" (2016).

Why is this breathwork style so forceful? The researchers state that "the strokes of continued exhalation in Bhastrika are aimed at completely emptying the air from the thoracic cavity. This yoga maximizes lymphatic emptying and at the same time, forceful movements over the abdomen due to diaphragmatic and abdominal muscles lead to further peripheral drainage" (Narahari et al., 2016).

Let's try Bhastrika—bellows breath / breath of fire:

- Sit in a comfortable yet alert position with a straight spine
- If you have a yoga practice, you can sit in Padmasana or Swastikasana and use Chin Mudra
- Close your eyes, if that feels comfortable
- Take a few diaphragmatic breaths
- Exhale forcefully through the nose, using your abdominal muscles
- Inhale forcefully through the nose, using your diaphragm
- Repeat nine more times
- Breathe slowly and naturally for at least 30 seconds
- Repeat for up to two more rounds of 10 breaths and then a 30-second rest period
- Take a few deep breaths through both nostrils before ending the practice

How do you feel after Bhastrika?

____

____

____

Bhastrika is similar to another pranayama practice called Kapalbhati. Bhastrika focuses on forceful inhale and exhale, while Kapalbhati breath is only forceful on the exhale, with a passive inhale. If Bhastrika pranayama is uncomfortable, you can try Kapalbhati instead.

The Institute of Applied Dermatology's "Yoga protocol for treatment of breast cancer-related lymphedema" also includes alternate nostril breathing (Nadishodhan) (Narahari et al., 2016). This practice is also called Nadi Shodhana. Nadi refers to energy channels in the Ayurvedic system of medicine and Shodhana means purification.

Let's try alternate nostril breathing (Nadi Shodhana):

- Sit in a comfortable yet alert position with a straight spine
- Close your eyes, if that feels comfortable
- Take a few diaphragmatic breaths
- Use your hand held in Vishnu Mudra / Mrigi Mudra—index and middle finger held at the base of the thumb—to help you close off each nostril when needed

- Close your right nostril with your thumb and exhale through your left nostril
- Inhale through your left nostril
- Close your left nostril with your ring finger and exhale through the right nostril
- Inhale through your right nostril
- Repeat this cycle for up to three minutes
- Release your hand and take a few deep breaths through both nostrils before ending the practice

How do you feel after alternate nostril breathing?

____

____

____

You might discover something interesting if you practice alternate nostril breathing at different times. The body naturally alternates the level of flow in the nostrils throughout the day. Israeli researchers state that "nasal airflow is greater in one nostril than in the other because of transient asymmetric nasal passage obstruction by erectile tissue. The extent of obstruction alternates across nostrils with periodicity referred to as the nasal cycle. The nasal cycle is related to autonomic arousal and is indicative of asymmetry in brain function" (Kahana-Zweig et al., 2016).

Yogic Breathing and Stress Reduction

Now let's look at some pranayama practices that haven't been formally recommended for lymphedema treatment, but have been shown to reduce stress. Our friend OM/AUM makes another appearance! Researchers from South Carolina in the USA found that a 20-minute breathing practice taken from the *Thirumanthiram*, an ancient medical text from India, reduced several stress and inflammatory biomarkers (Twal et al., 2016) . The protocol included OM/AUM chanting and thirumoolar pranayamam (TMP).

Watch one of the coauthors share pranayama practices in this video: https://bit.ly/ThirumoolarPranayama

Let's try the protocol!

Sit in a comfortable yet alert position with a straight spine.

Close your eyes, if that feels comfortable.

Part 1:

- Inhale deeply through both nostrils
- Exhale slowly while chanting OM/AUM
- Repeat for 10 minutes

Part 2:

- Hold your right hand in Vishnu mudra/Mrigi Mudra—index and middle finger held at the base of the thumb—to help you close off each nostril when needed
- Close your right nostril with your right thumb and inhale through your left nostril, silently repeating the phrase "I'm relaxed" twice
- Close both nostrils and hold the breath while silently repeating the phrase "I'm relaxed" eight times
- Keep your ring finger on your left nostril and release your thumb. Exhale through your right nostril while silently repeating the phrase "I'm relaxed" four times
- Repeat this cycle for 10 minutes
- Take a few deep breaths through both nostrils before ending the practice

(Balasubramanian, 2015).

How do you feel after this practice?

____

____

____

Does the world around you seem more vivid after pranayama practices like alternate nostril breathing? You are not alone! Researchers found that after practicing alternate nostril breathing, study participants had an improvement in "perceptual sensitivity" (Telles et al., 2019).

Balasubramanian has a website dedicated to this practice. Visit https://pranascience.com/.

More Pranayama Techniques

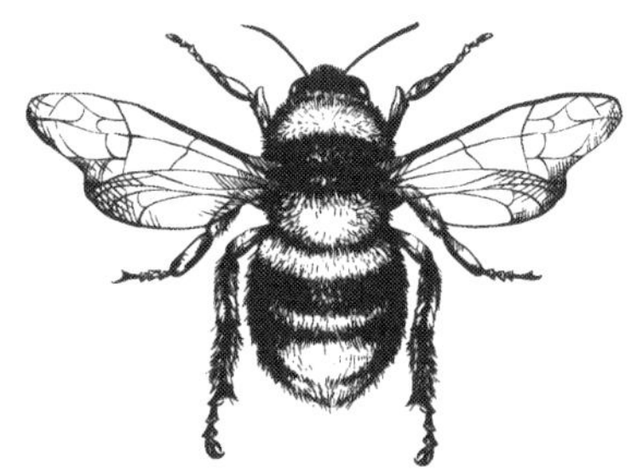

Humming

Many people enjoy humming while engaged in tasks of daily life. We can tell someone is having a good day when they are humming a happy tune! Can humming actually reduce stress, too? Indian researchers included humming in a 20-minute mindfulness protocol. Let's look at what they found.

The Society for Energy and Emotions (SEE) Protocol included:

- Five minutes humming
- Five minutes of breathwork - inhale for five seconds; exhale for five seconds
- Five minutes focus on positive emotions
- Five minutes focus on guided imagery for personal goals

(Trivedi et al., 2020).

What was the result? The SEE protocol resulted in a statistically significant increase in heart rate variability. The researchers say that their results provide a more active mindfulness option for meditators who experience negative emotions during more traditional forms of silent meditation. Researchers concluded that “active practice could be more beneficial to individuals with anxiety and depression as compared to silence and may have a positive impact on sleep quality” (Trivedi et al., 2020).

What about humming by itself?

Bhramari Pranayama is a special form of humming that encourages the meditator to hum so that vibrations can be felt in the face and neck. Researchers found that practicing Bhramari Pranayama, also known as humming bee breathing, may reduce heart rate and increase HRV and lung function in healthy individuals. One reason why this is happening may be “increased expression of nitric oxide (NO) and its impact on oxygen uptake” (Trivedi & Saboo, 2021).

What is the connection between humming and NO production? The paranasal sinuses produce NO, and the oscillating airflow caused by humming creates a dramatic increase in gas exchange between the cavities. In fact, NO increases 15-fold during humming compared with quiet exhalation (Weitzberg & Lundberg, 2002).

During Bhramari Pranayama we place our hands on our face and hum with our eyes closed. Closing the eyes and ears allows us to focus more easily on the humming sound and vibrations we are creating.

Let's Try Bhramari Pranayama now:

- Sit in a comfortable yet alert position with a straight spine
- Close your eyes, if that feels comfortable
- Close your mouth
- Close each ear with the tips of your thumbs
- Place the index fingers on the forehead above the eyebrows
- Cover your eyes with your middle fingers
- Place your ring fingertips alongside the bridge of your nose
- Place your pinky fingers on your cheeks
- Inhale through the nose
- Exhale a low-pitched 'hummm' sound at the back of the throat

- Feel the vibration in the facial region due to the vocalization
- Repeat this cycle for five minutes
- I also like to make a higher pitched hum that I can feel vibrating my nose

How do you feel after Bhramari Pranayama?

____

____

____

Researchers from India did a systematic review of the literature and found that Bhramari Pranayama practices have effects on the parasympathetic nervous system (Kuppusamy et al., 2017).

Conclusion

Why is working with the breath important to stress reduction?

When we are stressed out, sometimes it seems like we have a ton of thoughts and our brain is going a million miles an hour. How do breathing practices like alternate nostril breathing and breath awareness help calm our minds? Indian researchers found that pranayama practices like the ones we practiced earlier lead to "decreased cerebrovascular blood flow and increased flow resistance." They offer that "reduced levels of neural activity could explain the changes in cerebral blood flow." This is beneficial because "yoga breathing was originally intended to develop control over the mental state as a training for meditation and more advanced spiritual practice" (Kumar et al., 2022).

Breathwork may help in stress reduction because certain types of breathing can affect our body's sympathetic and parasympathetic nervous systems. We learned about the effects of breathing and the 0.1 Hz resonance frequency. We even tried several breathing techniques, including diaphragmatic breathing, alternate nostril breathing and chanting. Which ones would you like to incorporate into your daily self-care practice? Now, let's look at mindfulness and practices that work with the mind to reduce the impact of stressors on the body.

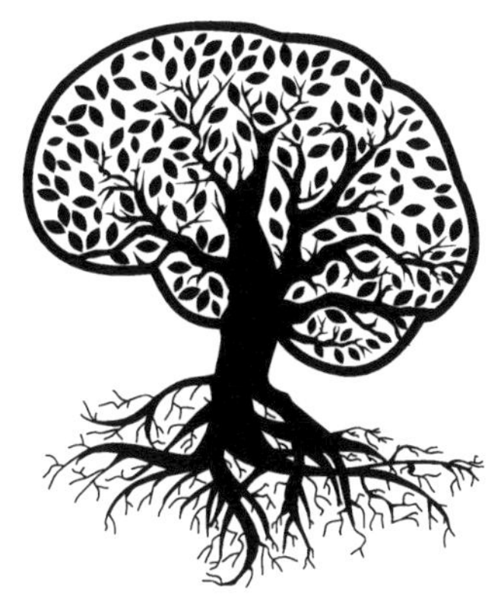

CHAPTER 4
WORKING WITH THE MIND

A nationwide survey in the USA of women with a family history of breast cancer found that African-American women were more likely to use CAM practices with meditation or spiritual components, comprising 45.9% of users. (Shani & Walter, 2022)

What to Know Before You Start

We just learned how working with the breath can be an effective form of stress reduction because our breathing rate has a direct effect on our body's nervous system. How can working with our mind help reduce our body's reaction to stressors? This type of stress reduction may happen when state (or dispositional) mindfulness leads to trait mindfulness.

Let's look at how mindfulness has been found to increase adherence to self-care and help with stress, mood and quality of life during cancer treatment. Then we will define mindfulness, look at some research and practice a few types of meditation.

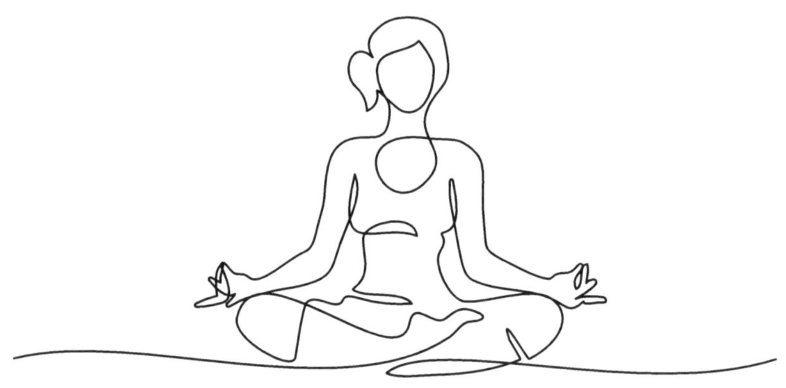

Mindfulness and Self-Care

Why is mindfulness important for those with chronic illness? I will write about its role in stress reduction in a minute, but first I want to share some interesting research. Daily self-care, including following doctor's orders and taking prescribed medications, is an important part of controlling one's chronic illness. Polish researchers found that three things “increase the likelihood of adherence with medication recommendations”:

- Strong internal health locus of control
- Higher level of mindfulness
- Lower level of emotional-stress coping style

(Bąk-Sosnowska et al., 2022).

Lymphedema requires extensive daily self-care. It is tough to have a lifelong, chronic illness. There is currently no medication regimen for lymphedema, but I have heard many, many stories of people who became overwhelmed in life and reduced their lymphedema self-care practices, only to see their symptoms worsen. People with lymphedema need to have a strong internal health locus of control—your self-care is in your hands! Increasing mindfulness may help make daily self-care easier to complete.

How else can meditation help? In “Clinical practice guidelines on the evidence-based use of integrative therapies during and after breast cancer treatment,” Greenlee et al. (2017) state that “music therapy, meditation, stress management, and yoga are recommended for anxiety/stress reduction. Meditation, relaxation, yoga, massage, and music therapy are recommended for depression/mood disorders. Meditation and yoga are recommended to improve quality of life.”

When looking at the research, I noticed that most research on people with lymphedema focused on treatments that would reduce limb volume, not stress. This is why I have included research on stress reduction that included people with a cancer diagnosis. Many people with lymphedema also have a cancer history. Interestingly, some research treats lymphedema as another "side effect" of cancer.

Let's Define Mindfulness

Okay, we've learned a little about the possible benefits of mindfulness. What exactly IS mindfulness? When someone mentions mindfulness, they can mean a few different things.

- Mindfulness can refer to a meditation practice itself, like silently focusing on an object and non-judgmentally returning focus to the object when distractions occur
- Mindfulness can refer to the state that is temporarily created during a meditation practice, like experiencing "non-judgmental, non-reactive, present-centered attention and awareness" while silently focusing on an object and returning focus to the object when distractions occur
- Mindfulness / dispositional mindfulness can refer to an "enduring trait that can be described as a dispositional pattern of cognition, emotion, or behavioral tendency"—when we become more non-judgmental, less reactive, and more aware in our daily lives after repeated periods of mindfulness practice

(Vago & Silbersweig, 2012).

State and Trait Mindfulness

State mindfulness is a term to describe mindfulness practices that can cause short term changes to mood during the practice itself. When practiced regularly over time, state mindfulness practices can result in trait mindfulness.

Being mindful isn't just another way to say "pay attention." If a person has mindfulness as a part of their personality, they have a tendency to accept thoughts, feelings and what's happening in the present moment without judgment or unduly fixating on one thing. Learning this was a BIG a-ha moment for me. Being mindful isn't just being able to focus or pay attention, it's the ability to place attention on something AND accept what's happening without judging, blaming or fixating on anything.

Research has shown that higher levels of dispositional mindfulness predict lower levels of self-reported pain in adults. Researchers from the USA found that, in people without chronic pain, having stronger dispositional mindfulness reduces pain catastrophizing which results in less pain. The researchers explain that "present oriented and non-judgmental awareness may influence the early stage of pain where the cognitive process begins, functioning as a precursor to pain catastrophizing" (Wilson et al., 2023). "Catastrophizing" is seen as a pejorative term, so I prefer to use the term "pain-related worry."

Let's look at a modern definition of mindfulness first, then we'll look at two examples of research that show improvement over time.

What is Mindfulness?

Jon Kabat Zinn, the founder of Mindfulness-Based Stress Reduction (MBSR), describes mindfulness as "awareness that arises through paying attention, on purpose, in the present moment, non-judgmentally."

What is Awareness?

When we speak about mindful awareness, we mean awareness in four different areas of our experience:

- What's happening in our body
- What feelings and sensations are present
- What's happening in our mind / our mental state
- What phenomena are arising in our consciousness

(Vago & Silbersweig, 2012).

This has definitely been the result of my own mindfulness practice. As I spent time paying attention, on purpose and without judgment, I started experiencing a greater awareness of what is happening in my body, of what my feelings are, and what's going on in my mind. It's good to be aware that this will happen—if you stop and pay attention, you may feel more of the feelings, sensations, emotions and mental states that are already present. Acceptance is the act of recognizing and allowing one's current reality. Mindfulness involves nonjudgmental acceptance of what is present in this moment.

Awareness of Breath Practice

Let's try a simple awareness of breath mindfulness practice now. The previous chapter was full of practices where we were focusing on breathing a certain way. Now, we will just focus on being aware of breathing.

- Take a comfortable position. Try sitting with your spine straight, if possible. If sitting on the floor, try sitting on a meditation cushion or folded blanket. Many meditators find it more comfortable when their hips are above their knees
- Settle in and get a sense of allowing the chair or floor to hold your body
- Close your eyes, or keep them open and gaze down the front of your nose to the floor
- Connect with breathing and find a place where the sensation of breathing is the strongest. It may be at the tip of the nose, where cool air enters and warmer air leaves the body. It may be in the belly
- Gently focus on that area and breathe naturally for 10 breaths

- If a thought comes, gently let it go and refocus on your breath
- After 10 breaths, wiggle your fingers and toes and open your eyes if they are closed

How do you feel after this practice?

____

____

____

Mindfulness-Based Stress Reduction

Mindfulness-Based Stress Reduction (MBSR) is an eight-week course developed by Dr. Jon Kabat-Zinn which includes seated meditation, body scan, walking meditation, yoga, and other practices that help reduce stress. Research has found that MBSR has positive effects on quality of life, anxiety, depression, mood, perceived stress, sleep quality, and fatigue (Reich et al., 2017). This class is offered online and in person. Let's look at the research behind this program:

Swedish researchers conducted a systematic review of systematic reviews for interventions following treatment for breast cancer and found that "mindfulness-based stress reduction intervention significantly improved anxiety, depression, stress and overall [Quality of Life]" (Olsson et al., 2019).

Researchers did a systematic review of 36 existing studies exploring the effects of Mindfulness Based Interventions (Mindfulness-Based Stress Reduction, Mindfulness-Based Cognitive Therapy, and Mindfulness-Based Cancer Recovery) on symptoms of depression, anxiety and cancer related fatigue in patients with cancer. They found that the mindfulness interventions were more effective at reducing anxiety and cancer related fatigue both after the intervention and at a follow-up at least three months after the program ended (Chayadi et al., 2022).

Research has also been done at Moffitt Cancer Center and Research Institute on the efficacy of MBSR(BC), a 6-week program adapted from the original MBSR curriculum and adapted to the needs of people with breast cancer. Researchers concluded that MBSR(BC) may help normalize pro-inflammatory cytokine levels and "clinicians might consider offering this program to survivors who want to stay healthy but are anxious about recurrence and often suffer from other psychological and physical symptoms" (Reich et al., 2017).

Find a list of MBSR instructors here: https://www.mindfulleader.org/mbsr-certified-teacher-directory

Find a MBCT Therapist here: https://www.psychologytoday.com/us/therapists/mindfulness-based-mbct

Let's take a closer look at different types of meditation practices. How can we work with our mind to reduce stress?

Focused Awareness Practices

In focused attention meditation, we are focusing on one particular thing and reorienting ourselves back to the focus of attention without judgment or negative reaction when distractions occur. This practice seeks to stabilize the mind. When the mind is not stabilized, we may feel "distraction, torpor, and hyperexcitability" (Vago & Silbersweig, 2012).

Distractions are a normal part of the practice. I like to explain the practice of meditation by comparing it to sports. In sports, skills are built by repeated practice. A basketball player learns to play by shooting and missing the hoop, catching the rebound and patiently shooting again and again. It's the repeated practice of returning to the focus of meditation without judgment or negative reaction that helps us become more non-judgmental, less reactive, and more aware in our daily lives.

Let's try a focused awareness practice that is used with people with lymphedema. The "Yoga protocol for treatment of breast cancer-related lymphedema" lists focused meditation on a candle flame, a practice known as Tratak, as part of their protocol, along with yoga asana, pranayama practices and focused meditation on the lymphatic system (Narahari et al., 2016).

Let's try Tratak now:

- Place a candle an arm's length from your seat, so that the candle flame will be at chest height
- Light the candle (you can also use a battery powered candle)
- Sit in a comfortable position with your spine erect
- Gaze at the flame for 10–15 seconds
- Close your eyes
- If you see the afterimage of the flame with closed eyes, concentrate on it until it fades
- Open your eyes again and gaze at the flame for 10–15 seconds
- Close your eyes
- Concentrate on the afterimage of the flame with closed eyes until it fades
- Repeat gazing at the flame and then at the afterimage for one more cycle
- Blow the flame out and bring the meditation to a close

How do you feel after Tratak?

____

____

____

Open Awareness Practices

In open awareness / open monitoring meditation, we are aware of any and everything but we do not get stuck in ruminating or focusing on any one thing. We can notice things we feel inside our bodies, things our senses notice (see, hear, smell, etc.) outside our bodies, and thoughts that occur (Vago & Silbersweig, 2012). Researchers from the USA found that an open monitoring mindfulness intervention resulted in "demonstrable changes in emotional processing indicative of reduced emotional reactivity" for novice meditators (Lin et al., 2016).

Let's try a 20-minute open monitoring meditation now:

https://soundcloud.com/ucsdmindfulness/20-min-seated-meditation-by-steve-hickman

How do you feel after this practice?

____

____

____

Loving kindness / Self-Compassion practices

Previous types of mindfulness focused on something in the environment and gently turned the focus away from any thoughts. Loving kindness meditation focuses on repeating phrases that seek to create positive emotions toward oneself and others. Let's try this exercise for two minutes. Begin by sitting in a comfortable position, and close your eyes if that feels comfortable to you.

First Minute

Think of a person or pet that is easy to love.

Silently repeat these phrases:

- "May you be happy"
- "May you be healthy"
- "May you be safe"
- "May you have ease of being"

Second Minute

Silently repeat these phrases:

- "May I be happy"
- "May I be healthy"
- "May I be safe"
- "May I have ease of being"

When you are finished, open your eyes, move your fingers and toes, and stretch.

Note: Loving kindness meditation is not easy for everyone. If the second part feels difficult or "fake," imagine a loved one saying these phrases to you instead.

How do you feel after this practice?

____

____

____

Self-Compassion Meditation

Self-compassion is the practice of being aware of our suffering and taking gentle action to soothe it. Living with lymphedema can be hard. You are human, so it is only natural to feel frustrated about your condition. You are not alone. Try this exercise for two minutes.

- Sit in a comfortable position, and close your eyes if that feels comfortable
- Place a hand over your heart, if that feels comfortable
- Say silently “It is hard to experience lymphedema”
- Say silently “This is part of being human; there is nothing wrong with feeling frustrated about my condition; I am not the only one’
- Say something kind to yourself (What would you say to a friend struggling with a chronic illness or chronic stress?)
- Feel your body against the furniture
- Open your eyes, move your fingers and toes, and stretch

How do you feel after this practice?

____

____

____

Were either of these practices uncomfortable? Researchers have found that people with higher levels of rumination may want to focus on other mindfulness practices first (Frostadottir & Dorjee, 2019). Rumination is the act of rehashing or dwelling on past experiences.

Why is loving kindness / self-compassion difficult for people with high levels of rumination or perfectionists? In my experience, many clients have a hard time being compassionate towards themselves and "letting themselves off the hook," and as a result may feel uncomfortable engaging in self-compassion exercises, especially if they do not believe they are worthy of such compassion.

Research suggests that for certain people, positive self-statements may be ineffective and detrimental; they have found that if people are allowed to focus on contradictory thoughts, along with affirmative thoughts, they are more equipped to handle stressors than if they did not combine these two actions. This may be especially true for people who unsuccessfully struggle to avoid negative thoughts (Wood et al., 2009). One option is to try saying kind statements while focusing on feeling both comfortable and uncomfortable with accepting them at the same time.

More Guidance on Adding Meditation to Your Self-Care Practices

Greenlee et al. state that most meditation practices have four elements in common:

- Quiet location
- Comfortable posture
- Focus of attention
- Open attitude of letting thoughts come and go without judgment

(2017).

I want to share some information on meditation I included in my very first book for my clients with lymphedema: *Swollen, Bloated and Puffy*. I'll share some tips I learned the hard way in my first few years of meditating.

Meditation for beginners will always involve thoughts, and they may be intrusive thoughts we don't want to think about. Meditation reduces anxiety not by ending anxious thoughts but by allowing them to pass—like a child learning to play catch with a ball.

Have you ever seen major league baseball triple play? The ball is in and out of the glove in record time because the players saw the ball coming and were able to recognize it and then let it leave their glove. If anxious thoughts are like a baseball, the goal of learning to work with the ball effectively is to not hold onto the ball.

Okay, so we'll get the ball out of our proverbial glove, you say. But first, let's consider another major meditation misconception. This one is about the best way to let a thought pass. Many beginning meditators believe that thoughts during meditation mean they are a failure and that "forcing" themselves not to think and berating themselves when they do is the only way to "win" at meditating.

Instead, we can let thoughts pass by recognizing and naming them ("thinking" or "this is anxiety") and returning to the breath. Name, return. Name, return. Name, return. Much like a player catches hundreds of balls during a baseball drill, this process can happen hundreds of times during meditation, and it is an essential skill to develop. The magic part for me is when the skill of recognizing a thought starts appearing in my everyday life. Instead of getting caught up in anxious thoughts, I can begin to recognize them when the first thought comes to mind and I'm able to label it before it overwhelms me.

Tips for Adding Meditation to Your Self-care Practices

Tip 1: Choose Your Space

The first tip is to select one spot in the home or yard to meditate and keep necessary items nearby—pillows, blankets, gratitude journal, etc. Meditating at the ocean or a canyon? Place all needed items in a bag and store the bag in a specific place so it's easily located.

Tip 2: Choose Your Meditation

Determine in advance how long and which meditation will be used. A meditation app can provide support for silent and guided meditations. Important: learn a lesson from me and don't shock yourself out of the meditation with a loud, annoying alarm. I have to admit, I used to use the alarm on the stove before meditation apps were created. Make sure the sound is soothing. In a pinch, use a relaxing song from your phone's music collection as the alarm.

Tip 3: Choose Your Reminder

Pick a "reminder" for your meditation, an event that happens right before it's time to meditate. That could be walking the dog, making a cup of tea, or returning from driving the kids to school. The event will remind you it is time to meditate and the location, supplies, time and type of meditation are already decided. All that's left to do is enter into the present moment.

My Space, Meditation and Reminder:

____

____

____

Once you have a regular meditation schedule, you might want to fit tiny meditative moments into the rest of your day. Here are five ways you can relax, no matter how busy your schedule is.

If you have five minutes, try a body scan. Sitting or lying down, find a comfortable position and gently focus on different parts of your body in this relaxing technique. Start by feeling your toes for two breaths, then feel each different body part, switching every second inhale. Breathe and feel the feet, ankles, lower legs and knees. Continue to focus on how your body feels from the inside of your thighs, hips, lower back, abdomen, upper back, shoulders, chest, arms, hands and fingers. You can finish your body scan by feeling inside your neck, jaw, face, ears and scalp, each for two breaths. Finally, focus on your entire body, breathing peacefully for a few breaths. This can be done first thing in the morning, at night in bed, or when you are a passenger in a car.

If you have one minute, focus on your breath. This exercise can be done at your desk or even in a tense meeting. Take a slow deep inhale through your nose, then exhale through your nose. Count to two, then inhale again. Pausing in between breaths brings relaxation.

If you are waiting in line, whether at the grocery store or for your morning coffee, take 30 seconds to notice what is going on in your body. With each breath, focus on relaxing the muscles around the eyes, then the forehead, then the jaw, then letting the shoulders be at ease.

Where do we feel tense in our body? Often, it's not just where we think. Try this trick: imagine you are making a business presentation and were just asked a question you can't answer. Feel that anxiety in your body. Now, notice what parts of your body tensed up. Your hands? Your face? Your belly? Focus on relaxing your personal list of tense body parts the next time you need a dose of relaxation. For me, it's in my chest and my hamstrings.

More About Guided Meditation

Guided meditation is a great resource for new and experienced meditators who would like more support for meditation practice. In this practice, a meditation teacher provides verbal guidance, offering prompts and letting us know when the meditation is completed. Apps like Insight Timer offer a variety of guided meditations. A great option for jumpstarting a meditation practice is to take a "meditation challenge." A meditation challenge is a program where a meditation teacher will choose a meditation each day for a period of time. If following the challenge makes you feel overwhelmed, simply stop the challenge.

One final tip: There are dozens of different types of meditation. If you find one you dislike intensely, finish out the meditation session and then try a different one in your next meditation session.

Self-Compassion and Body Image

Let's look at the relationship between self-compassion and body dissatisfaction. Body dissatisfaction is the cause of much suffering in women. The good news is research is showing that self-compassion may reduce body dissatisfaction (Albertson et al., 2014). This matters because researchers from the UK conducted a review of the literature on health-related quality of life in people with lymphedema and found that negative body image and low self-confidence in one's appearance cause people with lymphedema to change the way they dress. Participants in one study said that "their self-confidence was negatively affected by the cumulative effects of seemingly harmless comments about their swelling by others" (Morgan et al., 2005). Comments from others may also affect self-care. We met an older lady with a lot of upper extremity lymphedema in my Certified Lymphedema Therapist class and she told us she stopped wearing her arm sleeve when she went out in public because people would always mention the sleeve and her swollen arm.

How Can Self-compassion Help?

Let's look at the different aspects of the problem.

- Body dissatisfaction happens when we evaluate ourselves negatively

- Body shame involves judging ourselves as a person negatively because our body does not conform to society's standards
- Body surveillance is a constant concern with how our bodies appear to others

(Toole & Craighead, 2016).

Let's look at why self-compassion may help. Self-compassion has three elements—mindfulness, self-kindness, and common humanity.

- Mindfulness helps us notice our suffering in a non-judgmental way
- Self-kindness involves "care and understanding" versus "harsh judgment or criticism"
- Common humanity allows us to understand that "imperfections are part of being human and that flaws and inadequacies make one more (rather than less) connected to others"

(Toole & Craighead, 2016).

Researchers from the USA asked women with body image concerns to listen to self-compassion meditation audio recordings for three weeks to see if this exposure would increase self-compassion and improve body image concerns. The study involved 228 adult women, and mindfulness practices used included:

- Compassionate body scan

- Affectionate breathing
- Loving kindness meditation

Researchers measured self-compassion, body dissatisfaction, body shame, body appreciation, and contingent self-worth based on appearance and found that participants who practiced the meditations had significantly greater increases in self-compassion than those in the control group. The intervention led to improvements on six aspects of self-compassion:

- Self-kindness
- Self-judgment
- Common humanity
- Isolation
- Mindfulness
- Over-identification

(Albertson et al., 2014).

You can try the meditations in the study here:

http://self-compassion.org/category/exercises/

Optimism

Canadian researchers took a look at the effects of optimism vs. pessimism in life expectancy of patients with a head and neck (H&N) cancer diagnosis. The researchers found that dispositional optimism is linked to many positive aspects of quality-of-life in the 101 H&N cancer patients surveyed before treatment and three months after treatment. The researchers concluded that optimism predicts 1 year survival rates (Allison et al., 2003).

Researchers from the Netherlands had people spend five minutes a day for two weeks focusing on their best possible self. They found that this practice can result in improvement in the level of optimism and "people who were already high in optimism profited from the intervention to the same extent as participants low in optimism" (Meevissen et al., 2011).

The researchers had the participants:

- Think of and write down all aspects that their future best possible self should encompass—personal domain, a relational domain and a professional domain
- Start each sentence with "In the future I will"
- Construct realistic and attainable goals
- Focus on the positive rather than on the negative
- Write a personal story in which they put together their earlier statements in a detailed and coherent story
- Imagine this story for five minutes a day for the next two days

(Meevissen et al., 2011).

Would you try this optimism exercise?

Gratitude Journaling

The link between stress and cardiovascular disease (CVD) is well documented, so when I saw that gratitude practices had an effect on inflammation in people with heart failure, I wanted to learn more! Researchers from my hometown of San Diego, California in the USA share that chronic stress is linked to alterations in autonomic nervous system (ANS) function, and problems with ANS function often lead to worse CVD outcomes. Researchers put together a gratitude journaling intervention in people with asymptomatic Stage B heart failure and found that increasing gratitude levels actually decreased inflammatory biomarkers linked to adverse cardiac remodeling (Redwine et al., 2016).

What was the gratitude journal protocol? Let's try it! For the next eight weeks:

- Each day, record 3–5 things for which you are grateful
- Take time to remember the day and focus on everything that is a source of gratitude
- Personalize the list to your own experience
- Search for the little differences that happen every day, not just the big stuff

(Redwine et al., 2016).

Tips for keeping a gratitude journal

- Be specific: Focus on the details of why and how the things in your life inspire gratitude
- Go in depth: Spend a little time focusing on each item in the day's journal entry
- Focus on people as well as things: Remember to also focus on people for whom you are grateful
- Keep it simple: You don't need a fancy journal or a timer to start practicing gratitude journaling
- Make it a habit: Set aside a time and place to write in the journal if it's proving hard to adopt as a habit
- Don't make it a source of guilt: Feeling gratitude shouldn't feel forced or make one feel guilty or ashamed. Some of us were embarrassed by loved ones and called 'ungrateful' when we tried to advocate for our needs. Gratitude shouldn't feel manipulative

Expressive Writing

Some people may find expressive writing a useful way to put their deepest feelings about lymphedema on paper. Researchers from the USA asked 52 women with stage 2 lymphedema to practice four sessions of expressive writing and found that the exercise was more effective in improving quality of life when the writers had lymphedema for a relatively short period of time and were more optimistic. It's important to know that expressive writing may actually be detrimental to people who "initially avoided engaging in the coping process" (Sohl et al., 2017).

The research protocol was:

- Write about the deepest thoughts and feelings specific to lymphedema and its treatment
- Write for 20 minutes
- Write for four sessions, with 48 hours in between sessions

(Sohl et al., 2017)

Learn more about expressive writing here: https://ggia.berkeley.edu/practice/expressive_writing

Professional Meditation and Mental Health Resources

If you are finding any of the mind-based stress reduction practices difficult to understand or perform, taking an MBSR program may be a good first step. Enrolling in an in person MBSR program gives you access to a qualified meditation teacher who can answer most meditation-related questions and help you develop a habit of mindfulness. If you find these practices to be emotionally difficult, especially if they bring back memories of past trauma, it may be time to seek help from a professional mental health practitioner.

Conclusion

We took a look at how mindfulness has been found to increase adherence to self-care and help with stress, mood and quality of life during cancer treatment. We defined mindfulness and the parts of mindfulness that make it so valuable in stress reduction. We looked at some research and practiced a few types of meditation. I shared some tips on forming a meditation practice. We finished by learning about the value of optimism and looking at a few protocols for increasing self-compassion and gratitude. There are many different types of meditation. I hope you found a few that you are looking forward to exploring more deeply. Now, let's look at how we can work with the body to reduce the impact of stressors.

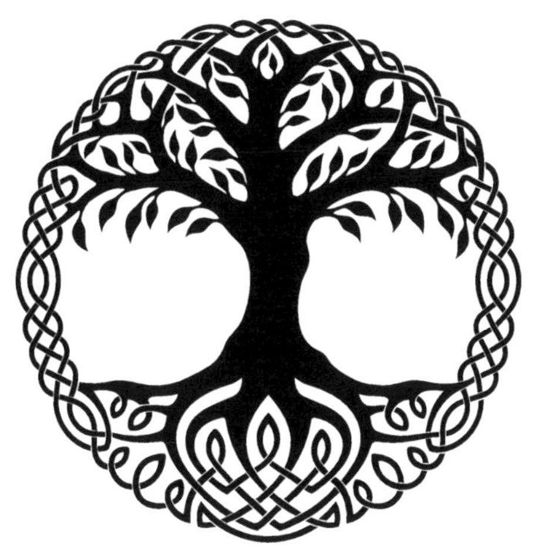

CHAPTER 5
WORKING WITH THE BODY

Working with Relaxation: Self-soothing Touch

How can we work with our bodies to reduce the effects of stress and put our parasympathetic nervous system back in charge? The simplest way I have found to work with my body is to place a hand over my heart. Let's try a simple evidence-based practice that is my go-to for clients who have just shared an emotionally charged story or experience.

I first reflect back the emotional content of their story or situation, to show them I was listening to them. I ask them if they'd like to see a practice that I use when I am going through a difficult situation. If they say yes, I invite them to place a hand on their heart and move it a little in a soothing motion for five breaths and repeat gently to themselves, “This is hard; it won’t be like this forever.”

Let’s try it now:

- Place a hand on your heart and move it a little in a soothing motion
- For the next five breaths, repeat gently to yourself, “This is hard; it won’t be like this forever”

German researchers found that participants “providing self-soothing touch and receiving hugs had reduced cortisol secretion responses to socio-evaluative stress with lower average cortisol values on three out of four measurement points after the stressor.” The people who used self-soothing touch were able to lower their cortisol levels to near-baseline after the stressor faster than those who didn’t (Dreisoerner et al., 2021).

Researchers encouraged participants to:

- Choose a way to touch that felt comfortable for them
- Concentrate on the warmth, the pressure of the hands, and their breathing

(Dreisoerner et al., 2021)

The researchers concluded that “self-soothing touch may not only be an effective option to reduce the effects of the stress resulting from the pandemic—for many, it may be the only option" (Dreisoerner et al., 2021).

How did that simple self-care practice make you feel?

____

____

____

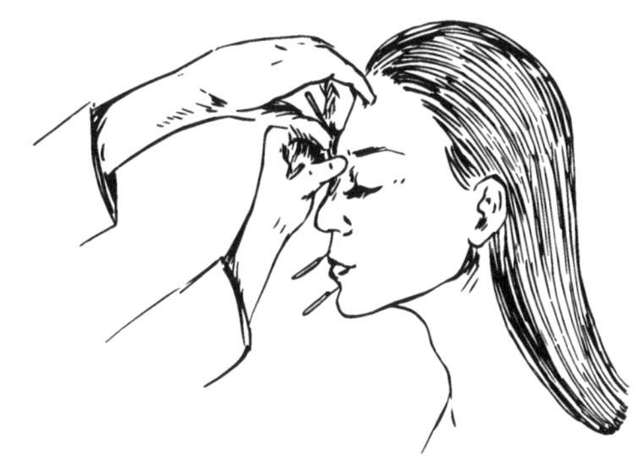

Acupuncture and Lymphedema

Acupuncture is a traditional Chinese medicine treatment that involves placing small stainless steel needles under the skin at specific sites on the body. Moxibustion involves stimulating acupuncture points with heat by burning Artemesia vulgaris (mugwort). When given by a trained professional, neither practice is contraindicated for clients with a lymphedema diagnosis (Valois et al., 2012).

Traditional Chinese medicine (TCM) theory states that the fluid stagnation of lymphedema is the result of damage to the meridians and collaterals and impediment of qi circulation from cancer treatments such as surgery and radiation. Acupuncture moxibustion therapy "has a positive effect on relieving upper extremity edema" and according to TCM, the treatment "can dredge meridians and regulate the circulation of Qi and blood by stimulating acupoints" (Jin et al., 2020).

Acupuncture is used on patients after cancer treatment, sometimes even right after surgery itself. Japanese researchers investigated the effects of acupuncture on two auricular (ear) points (Shenmen and Point Zero) and found that the acupuncture protocol affected heart rate variability and prevented postoperative agitation after colon cancer surgery (Arai et al., 2013).

Can acupuncture treatment improve quality of life and wellbeing in people with lymphedema? Researchers from the UK recruited people with lymphedema and a history of breast cancer or head and neck cancer and found that people with lymphedema can utilize acupuncture and moxibustion to address many lymphedema-related symptoms, even if they do not want needles used in the areas of the body affected by lymphedema. The researchers concluded that "acupuncturists and lymphoedema specialists can work together to bring about improved healthcare for cancer survivors with upper body lymphoedema" (Valois et al., 2012).

Brazilian researchers provided acupuncture to patients with BCRL and found that the subsequent increases in range of motion "positively influenced the wellbeing of the patients, permitting them to return to some of their daily life activities and reducing their feeling of incapacity" (Alem & Gurgel, 2008).

The points used were not on the parts of the body affected by lymphedema and included, according to Alem and Gurgel:

- CV12, CV3, CV2 – to regulate the meridian of systemic vessels, and lead to increased lymphatic circulation and hence a reduction in lymphoedema and lymphatic cysts
- LI15, TE14, LU5, TE5, LI4 – for the sense of heaviness, limitation of movement and pain in the upper limbs
- ST36, SP9, SP6 – for oedema, gynaecological disturbances, and facilitating blood flow

(2008).

Chinese researchers performed a randomized controlled trial of moxibustion on people with BCRL. In this study, moxibustion was used on the affected arm and the control group used a pneumatic circulation device. The researchers explained that moxibustion can reduce swelling and pain, and "the local irritation induced by this treatment can regulate the nervous system and improve blood circulation." Participants received moxibustion treatments for 30 minutes once every 48 hours for two weeks. The researchers found that moxibustion "relieves subjective symptoms of affected-side arm swelling, and reduces fatigue in patients with BCRL" (Wang et al., 2019).

Points used could include:

- Binao (LI 14), Shouwuli (LI 13), Jianzhen (SI 9) and Ashi points to promote the local blood circulation
- Waiguan (SJ 5)
- Shenshu (BL 23), the back-Shu point of the kidney.

(Wang et al., 2019).

Many people with a cancer history have added regular acupuncture treatments to their self-care practice. Research shows that there is no reason to discontinue acupuncture after a lymphedema diagnosis. Indeed, lymphedema symptoms may improve with continued use of acupuncture and moxibustion and protocols are available that can either involve or not involve the body parts directly affected by lymphedema.

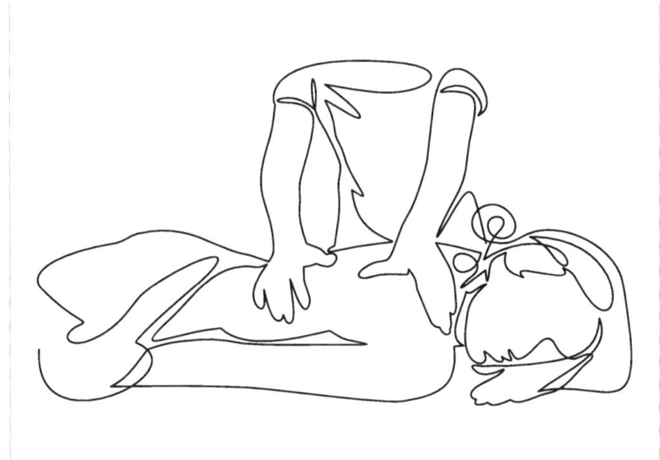

MLD and Stress Reduction

Manual Lymphatic Drainage (MLD) is a type of massage that supports the body's superficial lymphatic system. One giant misconception of MLD is that it only helps reduce swelling. This gentle, skin stretching technique can do so much more.

Let's take a look at what researchers have found about the health benefits of MLD.

Benefits may come from the effect of MLD on the lymphatic system, which in turn can interact with the nervous system. Turkish researchers state that "the autonomic nervous system is spread over many areas of the body and can be found in blood vessels, lymphatic vessels, and connective tissue. The lymphatic system and the hypothalamus work together to influence the responses of the autonomic nervous system" (Keser & Esmer, 2019). Sung-Joong Kim, a Korean physical therapist and researcher who has authored and co-authored several studies on this topic, concurs, stating that "autonomic nerves extend to all parts of the skin: blood vessels, lymphatic vessels, and soft connective tissue ground substance" (Kim et al., 2009).

MLD has an effect on hormones in the body. Inoue & Maruoka found that a 30-minute simplified lymphatic drainage session "decreased cortisol and dehydroepiandrosterone levels" (DHEA) in menopausal women (2017). Cortisol is a stress hormone and DHEA is used by the body to make estrogen.

Benefits may also come from the effects of rhythmic touch on the skin. An international group of researchers found that the non-MLD technique of "slow, pleasant brushing was effective in reducing pain perception" (Liljencrantz et al., 2017). Kim stated that "physical stimuli such as MLD can induce relaxation through stabilization of the autonomic system" (2009). Brazilian researchers conducted a literature review of conservative treatments for lymphedema and stated that by virtue of the techniques' use of superficial touch, "MLD can also promote:

- Quality of life improvement
- Sleep improvement
- Reduction of pain, anxiety, and other symptoms"

(Bergmann et al., 2021).

Pain Reduction with MLD

Other researchers have also found that MLD may have an effect on the experience of pain. Turkish researchers measured participants' pain levels before and after a MLD session and found that "MLD increases pain threshold and pain tolerance significantly in healthy subjects." They explained that rhythmic stimuli like MLD may create "inhibitions on the nociceptive receptors of the skin" (Keser & Esmer, 2019).

Kim also found a link between MLD and skin receptors. He states that MLD can:

- Increase physical immunity
- Accelerate recovery through body fluid control of dermal layer
- Accelerate recovery through removal of metabolites
- Increase emotional well-being
- Decrease sympathetic nerve activity
- Stimulate the dermis with abundant distribution of sensory receptors

(2014).

A long session is not required to see benefits from MLD. Kim also found that a 15-minute MLD session focusing on the neck region produced:

- increase of parasympathetic nerve activity

- decrease of anxiety
- increase in pressure pain threshold

(2014).

MLD and Stress—Not Just for Lymphedema!

MLD has also been tested in people without lymphedema. MLD can reduce stress in healthy subjects. Kim found that a 40-minute MLD session is "highly effective in increasing HRV and cardiac parasympathetic activity in normal subjects" (2009).

MLD has been found to reduce stress after breast cancer surgery. In one study, participants received a 20-minute MLD session after breast cancer surgery five times per week for four weeks. A Korean researcher found that MLD is "an effective method in reducing stress and pain in patients with postoperative breast cancer" (Ko, 2021).

MLD may even be more effective at stress reduction than other types of massage. Korean researchers investigated the effects of abdominal MLD on the brain activity of people with psychological stress. Subjects received either abdominal massage or MLD for 20 minutes. The MLD group experienced more acute neural effects that increase relaxation than the control group, who received abdominal massage (Shim et al., 2017).

MLD and Quality of Life

Greek researchers wrote a review article on the quality of life of people with cancer-related lymphedema and mentioned several studies that found that when MLD was included in lymphedema care, it improved quality of life for patients with lymphedema. The authors stated that "MLD in combination with physical exercise versus physical exercise alone has been found to further ameliorate patients' quality of life" (Kalemikerakis et al., 2021).

Turkish researchers conducted phone interviews to assess psychological conditions and quality of life in patients with primary and secondary lymphedema during the pandemic and found that those who reported that they "performed regular self-MLD and lymphedema exercises demonstrated positive effects" on the Lymphedema Quality of Life Questionnaire Arm or Leg (Begoglu et al., 2022).

The Role of MLD in CDT

MLD is one aspect of complex decongestive therapy (CDT). Researchers from the USA found that "gene expression of inflammatory markers can be reduced in lymphedema patients that undergo decongestive therapy" (Duhon et al., 2022).

CDT traditionally includes MLD and is the gold standard for lymphedema treatment. Kalemikerakis et al. looked at research on CDT and state that "patients who underwent CDT with MLD versus CDT without MLD . . . were found to have a noticeable enhance in emotions of wellness, lymphedema-related pain, weight and limb size, skin tension, sleep disturbances and skin infections." These findings were also found in research combining MLD with low-level laser therapy versus just treating lymphedema with low-level laser therapy alone (2021).

The authors state that "patients in the CDT + MLD group had a better quality of life, mainly in the physical and mental dimensions, in the role functions and in the reduction of the pain compared to the control group" (Kalemikerakis et al., 2021).

MLD and Stress Reduction for Lymphedema

We have just read a wide variety of published findings indicating that MLD can be used for much more than limb volume reduction. Kim recommended that MLD be used as "one of the manual therapies for stress in subjects with psychological stress" and noted that chronic lymphedema can cause lifelong stress, which can make the patient more vulnerable to infection. Kim concluded that treatment should focus on decreasing sympathetic nervous system activity and increasing parasympathetic nervous system activity (2014).

Progressive Muscle Relaxation

Is there a role for Progressive Muscle Relaxation in lymphedema care? Let's look at research on this type of stress reduction, then try it for ourselves.

Researchers from the USA provided The Breast Cancer Recovery Program to a group of people with BCRL and found improvements in arm flexibility, quality of life, and mood at three months. Participants in the intervention group watched a From Lymphedema Onto Wellness (FLOW) video and practiced relaxation techniques at home daily. Techniques included deep diaphragmatic breathing, progressive muscle relaxation, facial massage, and "low-to-moderate intensity, muscle shortening, gravity-resistive arm flexibility exercises . . . supplemented by imagery, natural scenery with flowing water, and background music. The exercises visually resemble tai chi or qigong but correspond to verbal directives and relaxation imagery cues" (McClure et al., 2010).

Iranian therapists evaluated the effectiveness of RCDT (relaxation plus CDT) versus CDT without the addition of relaxation techniques on women with BCRL. RCDT consisted of 15 minutes of progressive muscle relaxation before each CDT session. The researchers tested the participants and found no significant differences in anxiety and depression between the experimental and control groups at the start of the treatment, but recorded a significant difference in anxiety levels between the groups in the ninth week.

The researchers concluded that "the addition of this intervention to the treatment protocols used for highly-stressed patients with lymphedema is therefore recommended" (Abbasi et al., 2018).

Let's learn more about the Iranian researchers' protocol. Abbasi et al. added progressive muscle relaxation to their CDT protocol for patients with BCRL, and found that progressive muscle relaxation techniques "reduced the anxiety and depression scores and the volume of edema" in patients with lymphedema during both CDT and ongoing home care of lymphedema. The protocol consisted of contracting different muscle groups for five to seven seconds and then relaxing them for 10 seconds, starting with the head and ending at the feet (2018).

Let's try a similar protocol now:

Progressive Muscle Relaxation (PMR):

- Lie or sit down comfortably in a quiet area where you will not be disturbed
- Take a few deep breaths and close your eyes, if it makes you more comfortable
- Squeeze each muscle group for five to seven seconds, then relax for 10 seconds

- The whole practice should take about 10–15 minutes
- Scrunch your forehead, then relax
- Squeeze your eyes shut, then relax
- Scrunch your nose, then relax
- Purse your lips, then relax
- Tense all the muscles in your face, then relax
- Feel the heaviness of your face
- Tense the muscles in your upper back, then relax
- Feel the heaviness of your upper back
- Tense the muscles in your upper chest, then relax
- Feel the heaviness of your upper chest
- Tense the muscles in your shoulders by scrunching your shoulders up, then relax
- Feel the heaviness of your shoulders
- Tense all the muscles in your upper torso, then relax
- Feel the heaviness of your upper torso
- Tense the muscles in your upper arms, then relax
- Feel the heaviness of your upper arms
- Tense the muscles in your forearms, then relax
- Feel the heaviness of your forearms
- Tense the muscles in your hand by making a fist, then relax
- Feel the heaviness of your hand

- Tense the muscles in your fingers, then relax
- Feel the heaviness of your fingers
- Tense all the muscles in your arms, then relax
- Feel the heaviness of your arms
- Tense the muscles in your side body, then relax
- Feel the heaviness of your side body
- Tense the muscles in your abdomen, then relax
- Feel the heaviness of your abdomen
- Tense all the muscles in your lower torso, then relax
- Feel the heaviness of your lower torso
- Tense the muscles in your butt, then relax
- Feel the heaviness of your butt
- Tense the muscles in your thigh, then relax
- Feel the heaviness of your thigh
- Tense the muscles in the front of your lower leg, then relax
- Feel the heaviness of your lower leg
- Tense your calf muscles, then relax
- Feel the heaviness of your calves
- Tense the muscles in your feet, then relax
- Feel the heaviness of your feet
- Curl and tense your toes, then relax
- Feel the heaviness of your toes

- Tense all the muscles in your legs, then relax
- Feel the heaviness of your legs
- Tense all the muscles in your entire body, then relax
- Feel the heaviness of your entire body
- Know that you can repeat this practice any time to reduce the stress in your body
- Take a few deep breaths to transition out of the practice

Here is a 10-minute PMR practice video with audio guidance from Northwestern Medicine: https://bit.ly/PMRNorthwestern

Rhythmic Skeletal Muscle Tension

In a different study, researchers from the USA had participants sit in an armchair with their feet up and rhythmically contract their abdomen, arms and legs six times per minute (which they called rhythmic skeletal muscle tension or RSMT) for three to four minutes. Remember from the deep breathing section that this rate of six times per minute caused a resonance in the body's cardiovascular system? Well, they found that the RSMT protocol produced high-amplitude oscillations in blood pressure, heart rate, and vascular tone.

The researchers suggest that the resonance caused by the 0.1 Hz RSMT exercise is similar to the effects noted in research on 0.1 Hz paced breathing (Vaschillo e al.,

2011). This is great because some people experience anxiety when breathing that slowly, and could try rhythmic skeletal muscle tension instead.

Let's Try it!

- Sit in a comfortable yet alert position with a straight spine and legs extended out in front of you
- Close your eyes, if that feels comfortable
- Take a few comfortable breaths and settle into your seated position
- Contract your abdomen, arms and leg muscles for five seconds
- Relax for five seconds
- Repeat six times per minute for three to four minutes

How do you feel after this practice?

____

____

____

Yoga Nidra

Yoga Nidra is a stress management technique that uses guided meditation to bring the practitioner into a state of relaxation while still being aware of their surroundings. The practice involves accessing a "state of consciousness (awareness) that occurs between waking and sleeping, similar to the 'going-to-sleep' stage (hypnagogia)" (Pandi-Perumal et al., 2022). This practice is different from Progressive Muscle Relaxation and Rhythmic Skeletal Muscle Tension in that you focus attention on the muscles, but do not move them during the meditation.

Researchers who studied the effects of 20 minutes of yoga nidra combined with OM chanting found that the practice relaxed participants and had an effect on the hypothalamus, decreased sympathetic activity, and increased parasympathetic and beta brain wave activity (Anjana et al., 2022) .

The relaxation-meditation portion of the Institute of Applied Dermatology's "Yoga protocol for treatment of breast cancer-related lymphedema" includes 10 minutes of yoga nidra (Narahari et al., 2016).

A yoga nidra session usually includes the following steps:

- Preparing the body for the practice / getting comfortable

- Repeating a Sankalpa / personal resolution
- Body scan
- Breath awareness
- Feeling sensations in the body
- Mental visualizations
- Repeating the Sankalpa
- Ending the practice session

(Pandi-Perumal et al., 2022)

A practice similar to yoga nidra called Non-Sleep Deep Rest (NSDR) has been popularized by Stanford Professor Andrew Huberman. There are many yoga nidra and NSDR videos available on YouTube.

Quality Sleep

Research has found that people with lymphedema have “atypical sleep disturbances” which impact both sleep quality and their relationships with their partners (Ridner, 2009).

A study of 163 Saudi women with BCRL found that “quality of life and quality of sleep have significantly decreased in Saudi women with different stages of breast cancer-related lymphedema” and both get worse as lymphedema progresses (Tamam et al., 2021).

A scoping review found that people with lymphedema resulting from breast and gynecological cancer had increased sleep disturbance compared to survivors without lymphedema. Researchers also found that "lymphedema is a significant predictor of insomnia and is a risk factor for insomnia" (Bock et al., 2022).

Sleep disturbances may begin before lymphedema develops. Researchers found that most of the African American breast cancer survivors who participated in a study in New Jersey, USA reported "clinically significant sleep disturbance from before diagnosis through 24 months post-diagnosis." Lymphedema was one of the risk factors cited for sleep disturbances at two years after diagnosis (Gonzalez et al., 2021).

Some research on manual lymphatic drainage has noted improvement in sleep, but there are no quick and easy answers for reducing sleep disturbances. If you are struggling with nighttime swelling or finding a comfortable sleep position, ask your Certified Lymphedema Therapist for tips and strategies. If you are experiencing sleep disturbances, reach out to your physician for advice or referral to a sleep professional.

Conclusion

We started off our chapter on stress reduction utilizing the body with a self-soothing exercise. We then looked at the positive effects of acupuncture, manual lymphatic drainage, progressive muscle relaxation, rhythmic skeletal muscle tension, yoga nidra and the research on sleep disturbances and lymphedema. I was most surprised at the amount of research showing stress reduction effects of manual lymphatic drainage. There is also an abundance of research on acupuncture in clients with lymphedema, but it is not well known that acupuncture and moxibustion can be used by people with lymphedema. Some of the stress reduction strategies mentioned in this book may improve sleep, but I have not seen any focused research on sleep interventions involving participants with lymphedema.

Let's continue our focus on the body by looking at the interaction of movement and stress reduction.

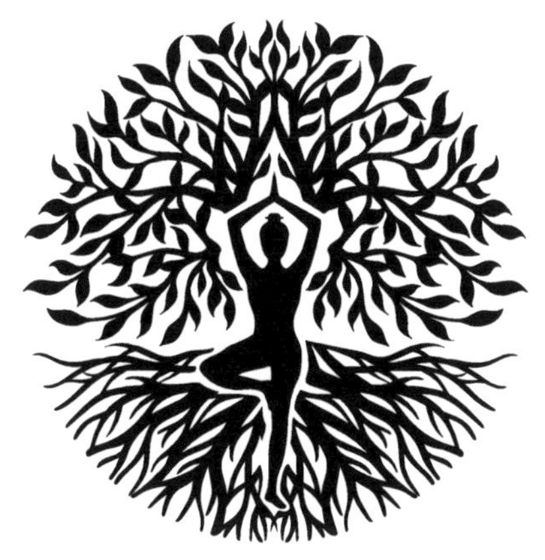

CHAPTER 6
WORKING WITH MOVEMENT

What to Know Before You Start

Many people with lymphedema have kinesiophobia, which is a fear of movement. Researchers from Turkey surveyed 74 people with lower limb lymphedema and found that they had both a fear of movement and impaired quality of life. Both were more significant in people with primary lower limb lymphedema (Sahbaz Pirincci et al., 2022). A separate survey of 40 people with lower limb lymphedema also found "high fear of movement and decreased physical performance and balance." Research has found that reductions in physical performance have both quality of life and psychosocial effects (Pehlivan et al., 2022). Researchers also found that over 47% of the participants in a group of people with BCRL had kinesiophobia and noted that “patients who develop lymphedema following breast cancer treatment often do not use their affected arms, due to the belief that their arms would become more swollen” (Gencay Can et al., 2018).

Concerns about excess movement causing an increase in swelling or making the lymphedema worse can result in kinesiophobia. Balance issues may also contribute to the fear of movement. Researchers state that having a balance disorder and a decrease in mobility can cause decreased quality of life. Balance may be affected by reduction in joint mobility, asymmetry between limbs, an increase in limb volume, and feelings of heaviness and fullness in the affected limb (Pehlivan et al., 2022).

It’s important to understand that you are not alone if you have feelings of fear around moving your affected limb. Exercising despite these concerns is essential to improving quality of life and physical performance. If you find it difficult to stick to an exercise program, enlist the help of a personal trainer or cancer exercise expert in your community. Your lymphedema therapist can suggest local programs. Other resources include:

- Livestrong program at the YMCA https://www.livestrong.org/what-we-do/program/livestrong-at-the-ymca

- Cancer Exercise Specialist Global Directory https://www.thecancerspecialist.com/user-directory/

Let's look at some basic guidelines for getting started with an exercise program. According to "Interventions for Breast Cancer–Related Lymphedema: Clinical Practice Guideline from the Academy of Oncologic Physical Therapy of APTA":

- Individualized programs of aerobic and resistance exercise should be provided for those who have BCRL (stages 0–III). (*Grade A*)
- Resistance exercise should be initiated at low level intensity and progressed slowly. (Best Practice)
- Individuals with comorbidities or complications due to cancer-related treatments should be referred to a specialist for evaluation and exercise prescription. (Best Practice)
- Sequential proximal to distal exercises incorporating diaphragmatic breathing should be used to improve volume reduction. (*Grade B*)
- Compression use with exercise may have benefit. (*Grade B*)
- Yoga may be a safe form of exercise but does not show evidence of effectiveness for lymphedema volume reduction. (*Grade C*)

(Davies et al., 2020).

Mind-Body Practices

Researchers from the USA looked at research on post-traumatic stress disorder (PTSD) and found that "mind-body interventions have a positive impact on quality of life, stress reduction, and improvement of health outcomes." They defined mind-body practices as "movements and postures combined with deep breathing," including practices like yoga, tai chi and qigong (Kim et al., 2013). Cross-sectional studies have found "an increased incidence of PTSD among cancer patients and survivors relative to the general population, with rates ranging from 5% to 19%" (Rustad et al., 2011).

How do mind-body practices work? Researchers state that stress-related disorders may occur because of "an imbalance in the autonomic nervous system (ANS), with over-activity of the sympathetic nervous system (SNS) and under-activity of the parasympathetic nervous system (PNS)." Mind-body practices may work by "normalizing the imbalance in ANS and increasing PNS activity" (Kim et al., 2013).

Researchers conducted a systematic review with meta-analysis of randomized controlled trials on the effects of mind-body exercises (tai chi / yoga) on heart-rate variability (HRV) and perceived stress and found "an overall large effect of Tai Chi/Yoga training on perceived stress. Four of the seven studies included in the meta-analysis demonstrated significant reductions in perceived stress." Additionally, they found "evidence for beneficial effects of Yoga on HRV is more robust than that for Tai-Chi" (Zou et al., 2018).

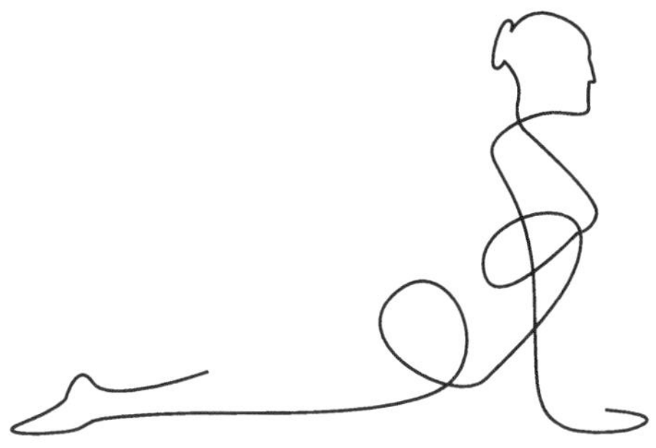

Yoga

"Yoga practices could potentially alter the expression of genes associated with inflammation and stress response." (Balasubramanian, 2015)

Does yoga influence stress reduction in people with lymphedema? Australian researchers state that "as a holistic practice, yoga may be of benefit by reducing both the physical and psychosocial effects of lymphoedema" (Loudon et al., 2017). Swedish researchers conducted a systematic review of systematic reviews for interventions following treatment for breast cancer and found that "exercise and yoga likewise have shown effects on anxiety, depression and [quality of life]" (Olsson et al., 2019).

What do people with a cancer history think of adding yoga to their self-care routines? Researchers from the Mayo clinic in the USA sent questionnaires to over 800 breast cancer survivors and 507 out of 802 respondents (63%) stated that they included yoga in their self-care practices. Almost 90% of respondents stated that yoga helped improve their symptoms (Patel, et al., 2021).

The most common symptoms that prompted the use of yoga were:

- Breast/chest wall pain
- Lymphedema
- Anxiety

(Patel, et al., 2021).

Interestingly, fewer than 10% of breast cancer survivors said that they had been referred to yoga by a medical professional (Patel, et al., 2021).

How might yoga be adapted for those with lymphedema?

Research published in the Journal of Lymphoedema adapted yoga sessions for participants with BCRL. Adaptations included:

- Avoiding heavy loading of the affected arm
- Restricting static postures

- Encouraging continuous movement
- Including breathing exercises
- Adapting floor-based postures to offer a seated or standing option
- Beginning with postures and movements that include clearing lymphatics of the trunk, then move distal to proximal in each arm

(Douglass et al., 2012).

In the "Clinical practice guidelines on the evidence-based use of integrative therapies during and after breast cancer treatment" document, Greenlee et al. state that yoga is recommended for anxiety/stress reduction, depression/mood disorders and to improve quality of life. Yoga may have positive effects on stress reduction because it is about more than just stretching or movement. They point out that yoga includes:

- ethical daily living (*yamas and niyamas*)
- physical postures (*asanas*)
- breathing techniques (*pranayama*)
- meditation training (*dhyana*)

The document states that "yoga is used for a variety of conditions, including stress, anxiety, depression, and fatigue, as well as a method to increase physical activity" (2017).

Yoga can also have an impact on the lymphatic system, if postures are used to stimulate the parasympathetic nervous system. Ryan states that "the lymphatic system, which is so dependent on body movements, benefits from yoga because of movement, but also yoga can control the autonomic stimuli causing the muscular walls of collecting lymphatics to contract" (2019).

Australian researchers created a clinical trial where 15 people with BCRL completed eight weeks of yoga according to the Satyananda Yoga® tradition, including:

- Breathing practices
- Physical postures
- Meditation and relaxation techniques

The yoga intervention focused on:

- Physical movements based on shoulder, spinal and whole-body range of motion
- Rhythmic stretching and compression of the arms, chest and upper back

The practice led to reductions in tissue induration of the affected limb and changes in quality of life, but improvements were not sustained after participants stopped the yoga practices, which suggests that the protocol needs to be a regular part of self-care to have continuing benefits. Reductions in tissue induration may have been a result of the combination of slow movement with slow breathing, which may have resulted in a gentle stretching and softening of the connective tissue in the upper torso.

Women in the trial reported:

- Improved well-being
- Increased awareness of their physical body
- Improved physical, mental and social functioning
- Transformative journey through illness

(Loudon et al., 2017).

Researchers from the USA ran a pilot study with six women with BCRL. Participants performed an hour-long modified Hatha yoga sequence three times a week for eight weeks, twice weekly in a live class and once a week from a yoga video. Researchers found that arm volume significantly decreased from baseline. There were no improvements seen in quality of life, and the researchers considered that this may be due to the small sample size and short duration of the intervention.

The yoga classes included:

- Meditation
- Progression of low-impact, modified poses, stretching and isometric exercises
- Poses focused on the shoulders, arms, and chest
- Breathing and poses to drain the lymphatic system

(Fisher et al., 2014).

The study's yoga protocol is available at: https://bit.ly/Fisher2014

Indian researchers conducted a systematic review of the effects of yoga therapy on lymphedema and stated that "it could be inferred that yoga intervention session of 60 min daily for a minimum of 8 weeks could produce beneficial effects in BCRL symptoms." Not all studies required participants to wear compression during yoga (Saraswathi et al., 2021). It seems that for yoga to work, it has to be practiced regularly as a part of ongoing self-care. It's a good idea to ask your lymphedema therapist for their advice on what type of compression to wear during yoga.

Researchers from The Ohio State University in the USA ran a randomized controlled trial on breast cancer survivors who had completed cancer treatment within the past 3 years. Participants practiced 90 minutes of Hatha yoga twice a week for 12 weeks and researchers found that "yoga practice substantially reduced fatigue and inflammation. Immediately post-treatment, vitality was higher in the yoga group compared with the control group. At 3 months post-treatment, the yoga group's fatigue was lower, vitality was higher ... more frequent practice produced greater benefits in fatigue, vitality, and inflammation."

The researchers state that "chronic inflammation has been linked to a spectrum of health problems including cancer, cardiovascular disease, diabetes, and osteoporosis" and concluded that "if yoga dampens or limits fatigue and inflammation, then regular practice could have substantial health benefits" (Kiecolt-Glaser et al., 2014).

Yoga Protocols for Lymphatic Filariasis and Upper Limb Lymphedema

The Institute of Applied Dermatology (IAD) in Kerala, India, uses integrative medicine to treat lymphedema, including the skin care treatments of ayurveda, yoga exercises, compression therapy and biomedical drugs for infection control (Narahari, 2022). The breathing exercises in yoga may help facilitate manual central lymphatic drainage and the yoga postures may facilitate peripheral lymphatic drainage (Narahari et al., 2007).

Breathing during the yoga protocol is diaphragmatic. Patients are asked to inhale during limb extension and exhale during flexion, with a longer exhalation than inhalation (Aggithaya et al., 2015).

IAD Yoga protocol for lower limb lymphedema: https://www.ncbi.nlm.nih.gov/pmc/articles/PMC4278136/

IAD Yoga protocol for upper limb lymphedema: https://www.ncbi.nlm.nih.gov/pmc/articles/PMC4959325/

Qigong

Qigong is a mind-body exercise with roots in Traditional Chinese Medicine (Fong et al., 2014). According to Memorial Sloan Kettering Cancer Center, qigong uses:

- Muscle relaxation
- Breathing exercises
- Meditation
- Body movements

(Qigong, 2022)

The practice is focused on the "internal flow of qi (chee), an accepted concept of vital energy force" and can create homeostasis of the body's parasympathetic and sympathetic nervous systems. Qigong may lower blood pressure and modulate urinary catecholamine levels (Qigong, 2022). Catecholamine are adrenal gland hormones released in response to stress.

The 'Clinical practice guidelines on the evidence-based use of integrative therapies during and after breast cancer treatment' state that, qigong is often used for:

- Anxiety, fatigue, and pain reduction
- Immune system support
- Physical and emotional balance improvements

(Greenlee et al., 2017)

Researchers from Hong Kong conducted a clinical trial and found that qigong exercise performed by people with previous training in qigong "could reduce conventional cancer therapy side effects such as upper limb lymphedema and poor circulatory status in survivors of breast cancer." How might qigong affect lymphedema? The upper limb movements of the "18 Forms Tai Chi Internal Qigong" resemble exercises a physical therapist might recommend for a client with upper limb lymphedema (Fong et al., 2014).

Many videos showing "18 Forms Tai Chi Internal Qigong" used in the study are available on YouTube.

Medical qigong "incorporates practice of coordinated gentle exercise and relaxation through meditation and breathing." Australian researchers conducted a randomized controlled trial of Medical Qigong and found the practice may improve quality of life in people with breast cancer and may affect inflammation and cognitive function (Oh et al., 2012).

Shani and Walter conducted an integrative review of mind-body interventions used by African-American cancer survivors (AACS) and "did not find any trials or qualitative studies that explored the relationship between AACS and other forms of mind-body exercise besides yoga, such as Tai Chi or Qigong," and concluded that this population may "not be aware of or have access to participate in other forms of mind-body practice" (2022).

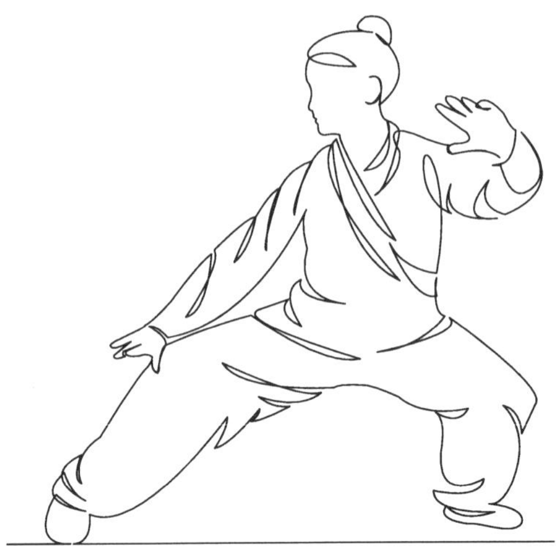

Tai Chi

Tai chi is a form of qigong. A tai chi form is a series of specific postures. Practicing tai chi may reduce stress and have an effect on BCRL if practiced as an ongoing form of self-care. Swedish researchers conducted a systematic review of systematic reviews of rehabilitation interventions following breast cancer treatment and found that "Tai Chi was shown to improve emotional wellbeing after breast cancer treatment" (Olsson Möller et al., 2019).

How does tai chi work to help people with BCRL? Australian researchers state that "a tai-chi trial that used a gentle arm opening and closing exercise for women with BCRL and reported a significant reduction in the tissue induration of the chest suggested that those actions may have reduced adhesions caused by fibrosis and improved the quality of the underlying connective tissue." The researchers suggested that the combination of slow movement and breathing may stretch and soften connective tissue around the pectoral and serratus anterior muscles (Loudon, et al., 2014).

The original article on the trial referenced above concluded that "forms of exercise that incorporate deep breathing and arm exercise, such as Tai Chi, Qi Gong and Yoga may also be beneficial for post-mastectomy lymphedema sufferers" and "may be useful as adjunct treatment along with CDT" (Moseley et al., 2005).

Many city and county governments or nonprofits in the USA offer tai chi classes at free or low cost to community members. Check with your lymphedema therapist for local resources.

More At-home Mind-body Exercises

Would you be interested in combining a simple exercise with deep breathing? Moseley et al. (2005) found that women with arm lymphedema who participated in ten minutes of standardized arm exercise and deep breathing experienced a reduction in arm volume, arm heaviness and tightness. The exercise is easy to demonstrate. Find details here: https://bit.ly/Moseley2005

Researchers evaluated a ten-minute self-care protocol for Japanese patients with BCRL which included:

- Japanese Radio Taiso (three minutes)

- Gentle arm exercises combined with deep breathing (one minute)
- Skin moisturizing care with grapefruit essential oil and sweet almond massage oil (three minutes)
- Central lymphatic drainage around the subclavian vein (one minute)

Radio Taiso is a popular calisthenics routine widely practiced in Japan, and research has found it improved quality of life in previous studies. The participants were advised to practice the Radio Taiso movements at half the usual speed.

The arm exercises were adapted from the Moseley et al. protocol linked above. The central lymphatic drainage and skin moisturizing took place during the patients' bath time. Researchers found an improvement in quality of life for those implementing this ten-minute protocol (Arinaga et al., 2019).

Watch a Radio Taiso video here: https://bit.ly/TheRadioTaiso

Labyrinth

> *"Most labyrinths in medical centers are primarily used to help reduce stress, manage grief, or relax."* (Davis, 2021)

What is a Labyrinth?

A labyrinth is a place for walking meditation. The word labyrinth is often used to describe a maze. A maze has many dead ends and is meant to confuse the walker. A true labyrinth has many turns, but it is one single path and is used for walking meditation. In a labyrinth, we can wander and explore within, without fear of getting lost on the path.

Labyrinths of differing patterns have been found throughout time and in cultures around the world. They have historically been used as a spiritual tool. The labyrinth pattern can be small and placed on a flat piece of wood, plastic, or other portable surface and the path traced with a fingertip. The labyrinth pattern can be larger and placed on a piece of fabric to create a portable labyrinth that can be laid flat and walked upon. The labyrinth pattern can be created from natural materials like rocks, constructed with different colored bricks, or painted on a surface to make a permanent indoor or outdoor walking space. In modern times, we can find labyrinths on private land, in community spaces, and at both religious and medical institutions.

Why have labyrinths made their way into medical spaces? Research has shown that labyrinth walking decreases psychological and physical stress (Behman et al., 2018). Walking meditation involves sustained awareness and "using the natural movement of the walk for fostering attention and presence, for being awake in the present moment" (Lizier et al., 2018).

> *"Walking a labyrinth can trigger contemplation, reflection, and transformation." (Lizier et al., 2018)*

What's the research behind walking the labyrinth?

A researcher from the USA conducted a literature review on labyrinth walking and found that labyrinths are commonly used for therapy in diverse healthcare settings, including cancer treatment centers and medical centers. People who walk the labyrinth report that doing so calms them, emotionally and spiritually, and helps them cope with their grief and make better decisions (Davis, 2021).

Brazilian researchers found that walking a labyrinth is a form of psychoneuroimmunology that can be used in integrative patient care. Labyrinths can be used by nurses to help patients undergoing oncology treatments reach a contemplative and altered state of consciousness (Lizier et al., 2018).

What may happen during a labyrinth walk? A recent study indicates that some people experience immediate physiological arousal while walking the labyrinth, while others experience a heightened physiological awareness and relaxation during and/or after a labyrinth walk (Behman et al., 2018). It is important to note that researchers found that the majority of people in one study reported emotional distress stemming from a feeling that the path was longer on the way out (Lizier et al., 2018). It is okay to step out of a labyrinth when you reach the center or if you start to experience emotional distress.

Rothlyn P. Zahourek, a certified clinical nurse specialist in psychiatric mental health nursing, stated that “although individuals did not consistently have a reduction in blood pressure or pulse rate after one trial, they did seem to feel better psychologically. Walking a labyrinth can also be presented as a type of meditation for people who find other forms difficult, who cannot afford formal meditation classes or training, or who hate to exercise in other ways” (2006).

“Labyrinth walking is an experience of irenic requiescence; expanding awareness; transforming potentials; and connecting to the beyond.” (Butcher, 2023)

A guide to walking the labyrinth from Roper St. Francis Healthcare: https://bit.ly/RSFHLabyrinth

Find the locations of labyrinths worldwide at http://www.labyrinthlocator.com

Exercise

We have looked at research on mind-body exercises like yoga and qi gong that can be practiced anywhere.

Now, let's look at types of exercise that feature aerobic or strength training.

Research has shown that exercise helps reduce the symptoms of lymphedema. Indian researchers conducted a systematic review of interventions for managing BCRL and found that "different types of exercises including aqua training, yoga, resistance, and aerobic exercises have been employed in mitigating BCRL symptoms" (Saraswathi et al., 2021). Spanish researchers state that "properly monitored physical activity and exercise is recommended" for both primary and secondary lymphedema including "both aerobic and strength training, on dry land or water immersion" (Río-González et al., 2021).

Exercise can also have a positive psychosocial impact. Chinese researchers conducted a review of treatments for BCRL and state that "participation in physical exercise during and after treatment for breast cancer can ameliorate psychosocial and physical conditions, resulting in active lifestyles with optimized survival."

The researchers also remind us of the potential for kinesiophobia after a cancer diagnosis, stating that "traditionally, patients with lymphedema or who are at risk for lymphedema tend to reduce physical exercise due to concerns about disease exacerbation" and remind us that research has shown that "exercise neither causes lymphedema nor worsens the disease" (He et al., 2020).

Water Exercise

Water-based exercise is recommended by many lymphedema therapists. Italian researchers performed a scoping review of the effects of water-based exercise on patients affected by primary and secondary upper and lower limb lymphedema and found that "water-based exercise seemed to improve pain perception and [quality of life] for patients with upper or lower limb lymphedema" (Maccarone et al., 2023).

One hydrotherapy protocol is named "HydroFE." People with lower extremity swelling attended two 50-minute sessions per week for a total of five sessions. Researchers said aquatic exercise is beneficial because "this medium stimulates both the neuromuscular and metabolic systems, positively impacting also the psychological side." They found that this intervention reduced lower limb volume and feelings of heaviness and increased ankle range of motion (Gianesini et al., 2017).

Find details of this protocol here: https://iris.unife.it/bitstream/11392/2354652/4/0268355516673539.pdf

Strength Training

Participating in a 90-minute strength exercise program twice a week for 13 weeks was found to positively impact participants' quality of life, including their perception of their appearance, health, relationships, and social functioning.

The weight training protocol was:

- Stretching
- 10 min of cardiovascular warm-up
- 'Core' exercises to strengthen abdominal and back muscles
- Weight-lifting exercises three sets of ten repetitions

For the first month, weightlifting was with minimal or no resistance. If lymphedema symptoms were unchanged after two sessions, weights could be increased by one-half pound. The exercises were:

- Upper body exercises included seated row, supine dumbbell press, lateral or front raises, bicep curls, and triceps pushdowns
- Lower body exercises included leg press, back extension, leg extension, and leg curl

(Speck et al., 2010).

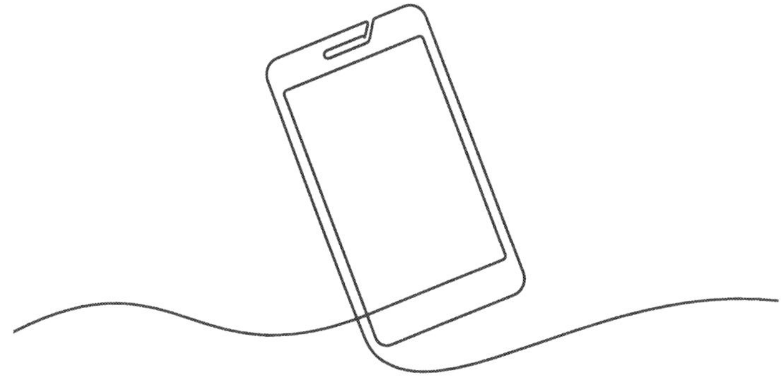

Digital / Smartphone

Spanish researchers looked at the effects of digital and interactive health interventions (DIHIs) on improving pain, anxiety, depression, quality of life, and upper extremity disability-related lymphedema in women with a history of breast cancer. Basically, these interventions are interactive video-based games. Play involves arm movements that may mimic exercises recommended for clients with upper extremity lymphedema and the game itself provides a fun distraction. The researchers found that virtual-reality-based therapy and smartphone app–based therapy help improve upper extremity lymphedema symptoms like reduced shoulder range of motion, reduced shoulder muscle strength, and handgrip strength, as well as helping with pain, anxiety, depression, and quality of life in breast cancer survivors

(Obrero-Gaitán et al., 2022). Specific DIHIs included Nintendo Wii®, Xbox Kinect and AquaSnap videogames.

Researchers from Saudi Arabia and Egypt had people with BCRL exercise with Xbox VR-based Kinect games five days a week for two months and the patients had a reduction in pain intensity and improvement in disability of the arm, shoulder, and hand (Basha et al., 2022).

Researchers from the USA investigated the effectiveness of The-Optimal-Lymph-Flow (TOLF), an internet-based exercise program for people with BCRL, and found that it had an effect on chronic pain, soreness, and swelling. The researchers concluded that TOLF "can be a better choice for breast cancer survivors to reduce chronic pain and limb volume" (Fu et al., 2022). Researchers describe TOLF as "an innovative and intelligent Kinect-enhanced lymphatic exercise intervention that teaches patients to perform correctly the lymphatic exercises." They state that this intervention resulted in "immediate effects on lymphatic pain, swelling, lymphedema symptoms, and lymph fluid level after a single training session" (Fu et al., 2021).

Find out more at: https://optimallymph.org/

Conclusion

We started the chapter off by learning about kinesiophobia, then took a look at how movement practices can be adapted to make them safer for clients with a cancer history and/or lymphedema.

We then looked at specific mind/body interventions, including yoga, qi gong, tai chi and walking the labyrinth. Each one works with the breath, movement and awareness of the body. Mind/body interventions are one aspect of a mindful lifestyle. Yoga, for example, is more than just holding postures on a mat. For the practitioner who wants to go deeper, yogic teaching includes ethical guidelines, pranayama, and mindfulness practices that don't have to involve sweating on a yoga mat. Qi gong is an energy practice that works with the body's life force. Labyrinth walking may be used for contemplation and prayer.

We then looked at protocols for gym-based exercise for people with lymphedema, including aquatic exercise and weightlifting. We ended the chapter by looking at digital interventions that use games to provide a fun distraction and mimic physical therapy exercises that can improve lymphedema symptoms. Now, let's look at how we can work with our senses to reduce stress.

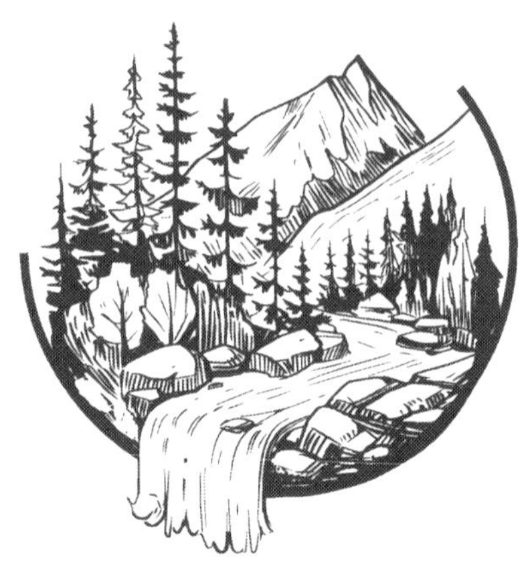

CHAPTER 7
WORKING WITH THE SENSES

Sense-based self-care

Have you ever used one (or more) of your senses to make you feel calmer and more "grounded" when you felt overwhelmed? The University of Rochester Medical Center's Behavioral Health Partners blog offers a quick practice for reducing anxious thoughts. Let's try it now.

- Start with a few slow, deep, long breaths
- Notice **FIVE** things you see around you
- Notice **FOUR** things you can touch. You can touch them, if you like

- Notice **THREE** things you can hear, inside or outside of your body
- Notice **TWO** things you can smell
- Notice **ONE** thing you can taste. It could be chewing gum, a drink or something else (Smith, 2018).

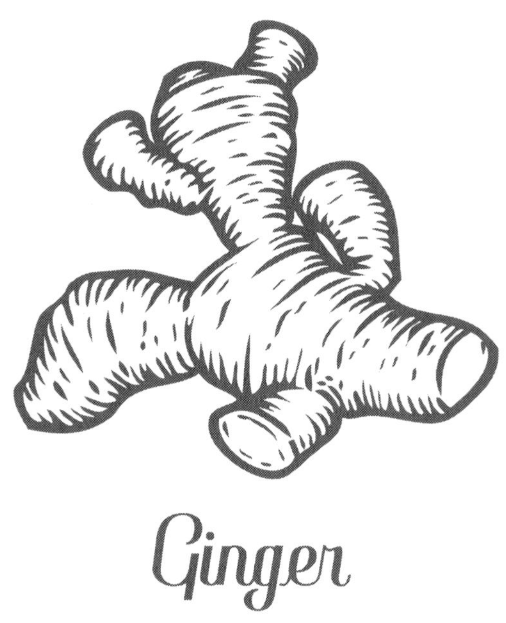

Ginger

This practice can be used any time and any place to help reorient us to the present moment. Here are some more examples of grounding practices that use our senses to allow us to reconnect with our bodies and provide us a sense of safety and connection. Which ones appeal to you?

Sight:

- Look at a nature scene, film or photo (Beukeboom et al., 2012; Levi, 1965)
- Read poetry (Davies, 2018; Delamerced et al., 2021) or sacred texts
- Spend a few minutes in sunlight (Beecher et al., 2016)

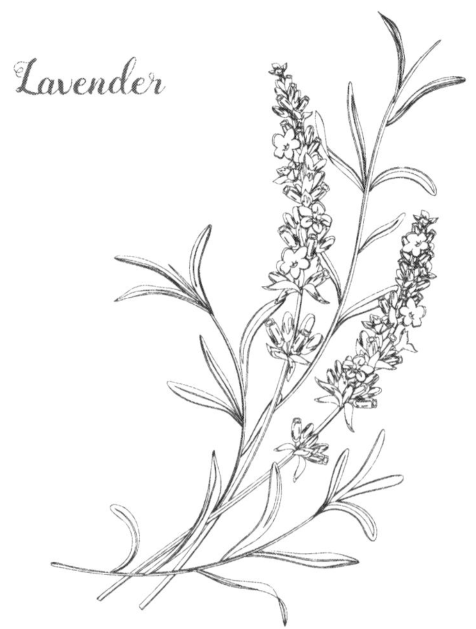

Sound:

- Listen to sounds in the environment
- Listen to soothing music, like the song Weightless by Marconi Union (Graff et al., 2019)

- Listen to binaural beats or 432 Hz tuned music for 10 minutes (Chaieb et al., 2015; Menziletoglu et al., 2021; Padmanabhan et al., 2005; Zampi, 2016)
- Listen to Tibetan singing bowls (Rio-Alamos et al., 2023)
- Listen to birdsong (Zhao et al., 2020)
- Listen to ASMR videos (Eid et al., 2022)

Smell

- Use essential oils / aromatherapy (Farrar & Farrar, 2020; Lizarraga-Valderrama, 2021; Wilkinson et al., 2007)

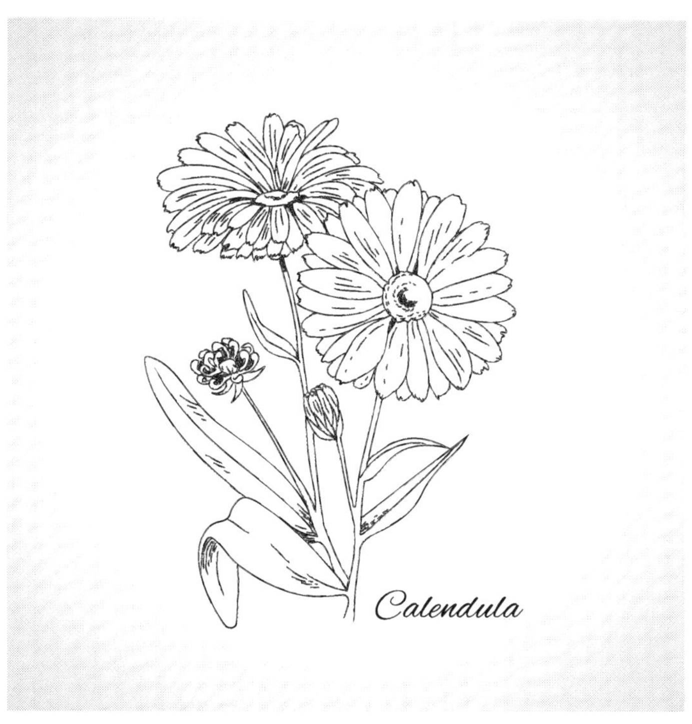

Touch

- Sit or lie under a weighted blanket (Vinson et al., 2020)
- Stroke a pet or a horse (Ein et al., 2018)
- Draw or color mandalas (Henderson et al., 2007; Khodabakhshi-Koolaee & Darestani-Farahani, 2020)
- Receive massage (Greenlee et al., 2014)—find a therapist at https://www.s4om.org/

Vestibular

- Rock in a rocking chair (Cross et al., 2018; Snyder et al., 2001)

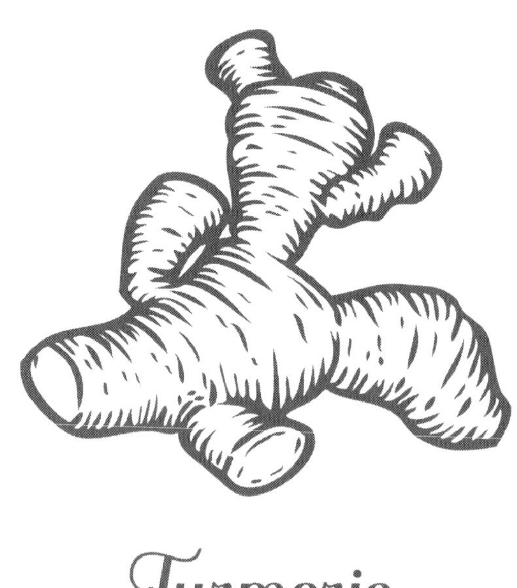

Turmeric

I hope this short list inspired you to think of other ways that you use your senses to relax and reduce stress. You can write them here now:

____

____

____

____

Time in Nature

Take a few moments to remember a day where you spent quality time in a natural place. How did spending time in nature make you feel? Research has shown a link between time in green spaces and a reduction in salivary cortisol, a physiological marker of stress (Twohig-Bennett & Jones, 2018).

What are some stress-reducing suggestions for spending time outside?

One type of nature therapy is time spent experiencing the forest with the senses, which is called shinrin-yoku, or forest bathing. Researchers from the UK explain that in this practice, we can sit or lie down in the forest and breathe in the phytoncides (volatile organic compounds with antibacterial properties) released by trees (Twohig-Bennett & Jones, 2018).

Chinese researchers found that the forest bathing model advocates for subhealthy people and sick people to spend time in the forest engaging in activities that generate a healing effect through forest environmental factors. Subhealth is defined as a state between health and disease, with symptoms such as fatigue, poor sleep quality, forgetfulness, and physical pain (Wen et al., 2019).

Does spending time taking care of your garden seem to help relieve stress? Horticultural therapy is designed for people with diseases caused by mental stress and focuses on hand-brain coordination and contact with nature. Sessions involve going into a natural environment to talk with others, make crafts. and garden (Wen et al., 2019).

Passionflower

Passiflora incarnata

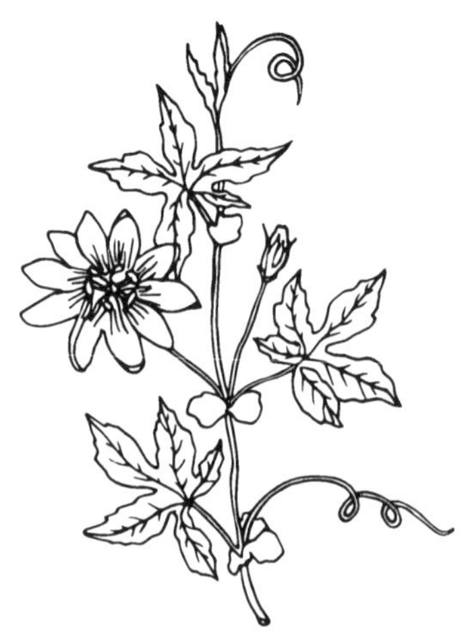

Researchers from the USA found that time spent in nature has many health benefits, including:

- decreased blood pressure
- decreased stress levels
- enhanced immune system function
- decreased depression
- overall wellness

(Mitten et al., 2016)

How can we make it easier for those who have trouble getting around to access nature in the USA? Ashley Matheny gave me some great advice at a conference a few years ago. She suggested that "if you look for 'accessible fishing' you can find areas that are easy to be near the water and often have a bench." More information about accessible fishing piers and platforms is here: https://bit.ly/fishingpiers

American Horticultural Therapy Association (USA): https://www.ahta.org/

Find local parks https://parkrxamerica.org/

Improving Urban Health Through Green Space

https://www.usda.gov/media/blog/2017/11/28/improving-urban-health-through-green-space

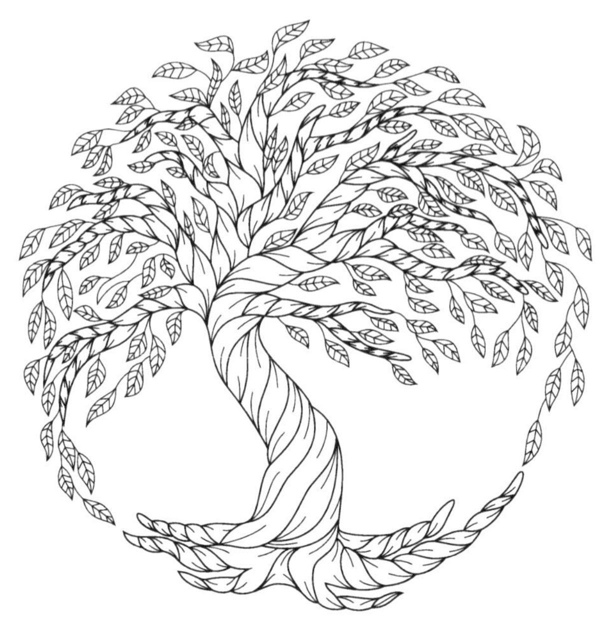

What About Our "Sense" of Humor?

Could utilizing our sense of humor help quality of life? Japanese researchers found that "patients with primary lymphedema have problems in health perception, discomfort, usual activities, and anxiety/depression." The researchers found that "coping with humor has a positive association with the mental aspect of [health-related quality of life] among patients with primary lymphedema contrary to dysfunctional coping such as denial, substance use, and self-blame, which are generally regarded as negative factors" (Okajima et al., 2013).

USA researchers conducted a review of the evidence on how humor influences physiological and psychological well-being and found that "laughter leads to episodes of sharply sporadic deep breathing" and that "various muscle groups are activated for periods of seconds at a time, while the period immediately after the laugh leads to general muscle relaxation. This post-laughter relaxation can last up to 45 minutes." They also cited research that found that laughter reduced serum cortisol in people watching a humorous video (Bennett & Lengacher, 2008).

One option is a practice called Laughter Yoga.

Laughter is a type of breathing characterized by strong inhalations and exhalations. Both breathing volume and respiration are increased versus normal breathing. The practice of Laughter Yoga was created by Dr. Madan Kataria and involves "simulated laughter interspersed with deep yogic breathing" (Meier et al., 2021).

Can Laughter Yoga reduce stress? German and Canadian researchers tested laughter yoga and relaxation breathing to see if either had an effect on the body's autonomic, endocrine or psychological response to a subsequent stressful situation. They found that laughter yoga did not change whether the participant experienced a situation as stressful, but it did affect the body's endocrine response to the stressful situation.

The researchers had a very interesting theory as to why laughter yoga might work in this way. The experience of laughing may reduce self-awareness and self-attention, which would result in feeling less shame during a stressful event. Shame may happen when there is a negative evaluation of our social self and experiencing shame may affect the level of cortisol the body releases. The researchers concluded that laughter yoga can reduce the cortisol response to acute stress (Meier et al., 2021).

Body Esteem and Trait Shame

Researchers from the USA state that body esteem levels and chronic shame can activate the hypothalamic–pituitary–adrenal (HPA) axis and result in the secretion of cortisol. Body esteem is "how one views one's body and appearance," and the researchers found that "participants who reported dissatisfaction with their bodies also reported higher levels of trait shame" (Lupis et al., 2016).

The researchers state that the "Social Self Preservation Theory suggests that the HPA axis is most likely activated in situations that threaten the 'social self,' potentially lowering self-esteem, social status, and personal worth. These threats to the social self are then proposed to elicit shame, which, in turn, activates the HPA axis" (Lupis et al., 2016).

How does Laughter Help Health Outcomes?

Researchers from the USA state that laughing can reduce muscle tension, increase cardio-respiratory system and decrease stress hormones including cortisol. Decreasing cortisol is important because cortisol is immunosuppressive and laughter could decrease levels of this stress hormone (Bennett & Lengacher, 2008).

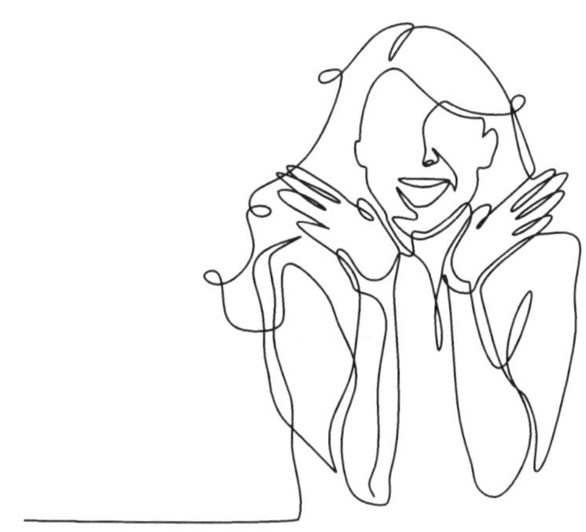

Laughter Yoga and Cancer

In the Initiative On Smile And CAncer (iOSACA) randomized controlled trial, Japanese researchers found that laughter therapy, including laughter yoga, reduced pain and improved some aspects of quality of life in people with cancer (Morishima et al., 2019). Korean researchers found that a "therapeutic laughter program was effective after only a single session in reducing anxiety, depression, and stress in breast cancer patients, [and] it could be recommended as a first-line complementary/alternative therapy" (Kim et al., 2015).

The supplementary material section offers a detailed description of the Korean laughter intervention: https://www.ncbi.nlm.nih.gov/pmc/articles/PMC4439472/

Try an online Laughter Yoga session here: https://www.laughteryoga.org/zoom-laughter-club/

Conclusion

In this chapter we tried a quick practice that used a check-in with five senses to calm our nervous system, then looked at the stress reduction effects of practices that specifically involve the senses. We then focused on the benefits of spending time in nature, and ended with a look at our "sense" of humor.

Now, let's look at the benefits of working with the community. We will revisit many of the stressors mentioned in the beginning of the book.

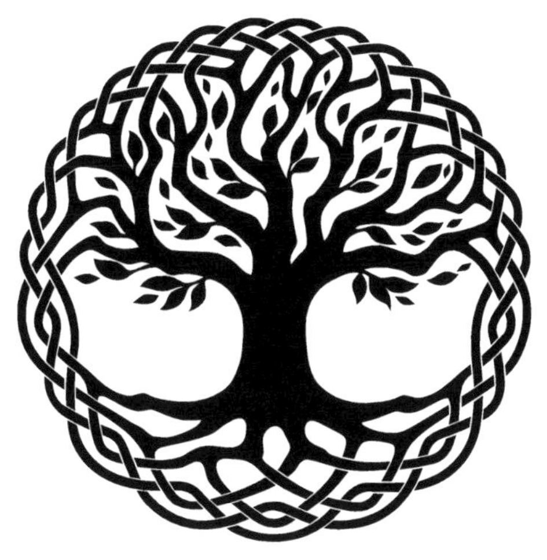

CHAPTER 8

WORKING WITH THE COMMUNITY

Fostering a sense of community and connection

Remember earlier in the book when I mentioned two ways to reduce the burden of stressors on your body? We can reduce the number of stressful situations and we can increase our capacity to handle those stressful situations. The practices I have shared so far have been aimed at increasing our capacity to handle stressful situations. But it is equally important to work together as a community and advocate for the reduction of many of the situations which cause stress to people with lymphedema. Let's talk about those situations now.

Researchers from the USA conducted a systematic review of literature on the psychosocial impact of lymphedema and found that people experienced:

- Marginalization
- Perceived social abandonment
- Social isolation
- Public insensitivity
- Financial burden
- Unsupportive work environment

Feelings of marginalization included frustration with "healthcare providers' or family's relegation of lymphedema as unimportant or trivial, and when healthcare providers provided conflicting, minimal, or no lymphedema information" (Fu et al., 2012). Health professionals and other experts must work to improve lymphedema awareness across all areas of medicine.

We can reduce perceptions of social abandonment and isolation by increasing awareness and connection. Connecting with others and feeling community are important to living well with lymphedema. Researchers from the USA explored the experiences of people with non-cancer-related lymphedema and found that "for many participants, meeting with a psychologist, as well as hearing the stories of fellow patients, was an important aspect of their inpatient treatment."

One individual shared, “knowing there were others that had the same problem and were going through the same type of struggle that I was made a big difference because I felt I wasn’t alone anymore.” Another participant stated that prior to talking with a psychologist and others with lymphedema, “I knew it could get real serious, but I didn’t know there was a way you could cope with it and live with it.”

Talking to others with lymphedema at the hospital “gave me hope it would be okay,” reported one individual, who described feeling “overwhelmed” when she first started her inpatient treatment (Bogan et al., 2007).

Researchers from the UK who focused on the lived experiences of men with lymphedema found that being diagnosed with lymphedema can have a negative impact on men.

- They need to meet other men with lymphedema but when men attend support groups, they may come away thinking that lymphedema is an old person’s disease because, in their words, “You go to the support group . . . [and] they are all elderly men”
- Men with head and neck lymphedema may also avoid recreational activities if they feel that their bodily swelling affects their strength and thus their feelings of manhood or their facial swelling affects their masculinity

Understanding of these issues is critical to men with lymphedema, who often benefit from access to knowledgeable healthcare professionals, peer support and self-care reminders (Cooper-Stanton et al., 2022).

Researchers from the USA found that "Latinas and their caregivers often report having more unmet needs regarding information and psychological support during and after cancer treatment than do non-Latina whites." The researchers' intervention acknowledged the importance of family and close friends (familism) and included "informal" caregivers chosen by the participants. Both the survivors and their caregivers experience psychosocial stressors during the survivorship journey and may derive mutual benefit from stress reduction (Badger et al., 2019).

Researchers from the USA conducted focus groups of African-American breast cancer survivors and caregivers and found that study participants experienced:

- A culture that discourages discussion of cancer, hence creating a cultural silence regarding diagnosis
- Lack of support services for African-American cancer survivors
- Lack of support services for cancer caregivers, such as coping strategies to balance work-life-caregiver demands
- Need for culturally appropriate cancer resources
- Need for a strong social support network

(Haynes-Maslow et al., 2015).

Research shows that "African-American cancer survivors have cited faith, family and friends, as well as church members as key sources of support." Caregivers are usually spouses, children, and friends (Haynes-Maslow et al., 2015).

Researchers in Nepal recommend that health workers emphasize the importance of social participation for those affected by lymphatic filariasis, a parasitic disease that impacts the lymphatic system (Adhikari et al., 2015). Ethiopian researchers found that "in a qualitative study among podoconiosis, leprosy, and lymphatic filariasis patients, participants reports that they mostly relied on their children and spouses for support. They had got psychological and economical support, taking over household issues such as cooking and washing clothes" (Abebaw et al., 2022).

Participating in community-based programs may improve health-related quality of life (HRQoL). Ethiopian researchers performed a community-based cross-sectional study on people with podoconiosis and found that "overall HRQoL of the study participants was higher than a study conducted in North Ethiopia. In the study area there is implementation of community-based podoconiosis prevention and treatment programs; this might be the possible justification of the differences" (Abebaw et al., 2022).

"Active coping strategies included engaging in selfcare behaviors (e.g. not putting strain on the affected arm), using medical equipment as recommended, and attending support groups and medical appointments regularly. For instance, a participant engaged in several activities to help manage BCRL: 'I have become more spiritual, involved in church, reading, I listen to music, and do yoga.'" (Buki et al., 2021)

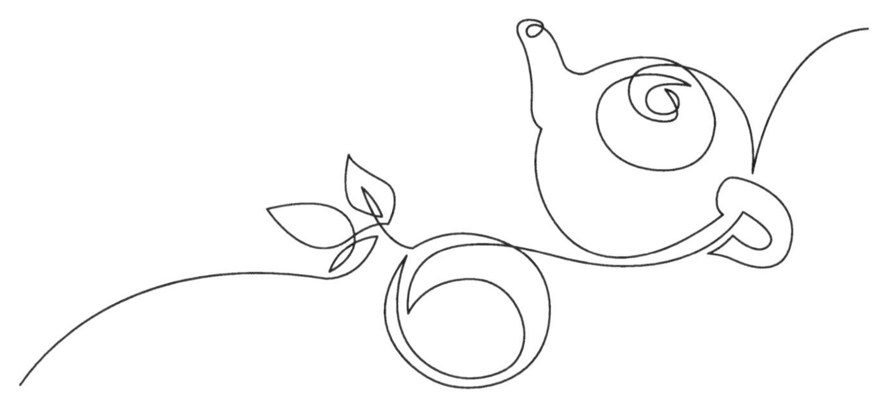

Community and Self-Efficacy

Nurses know that a lack of support from loved ones is a barrier to a patient's self-efficacy. An article by Farley published in the journal Nursing Open states that "social connectedness and support produce greater self-efficacy" and "interventions are limited in some patients when the family is opposed to change or do not support the patient" (2020).

What is self-efficacy?

Self-efficacy can improve quality of life and enable people to more effectively manage their chronic disease. Farley states that self-efficacy is "a cognitive process where, through environmental influence and social influence, individuals learn new behaviours that affect their ability to improve future events." Why is community such an important part of self-care? Farley states that "several reviewed articles identified a lack of support, either formal or informal, being a barrier to self-efficacy and positive patient outcomes" (Farley, 2020).

Reading and Writing in Community

Canadian researchers state that creative engagement "contributes to good health and well-being." They found that participants in a community-based workshop with breast cancer survivors reacted favorably to the program and felt it addressed their survivorship concerns. Two daylong events took place two weeks apart and featured a writing intervention (journaling). The researchers concluded that "arts-based interventions can enhance well-being in cancer survivors" (Thomas et al., 2017).

Participants in a shared reading group for people with a cancer history in Norway found that the experience helped them "balance life and cancer," and "disconnect" from their illness (Andersen, 2022).

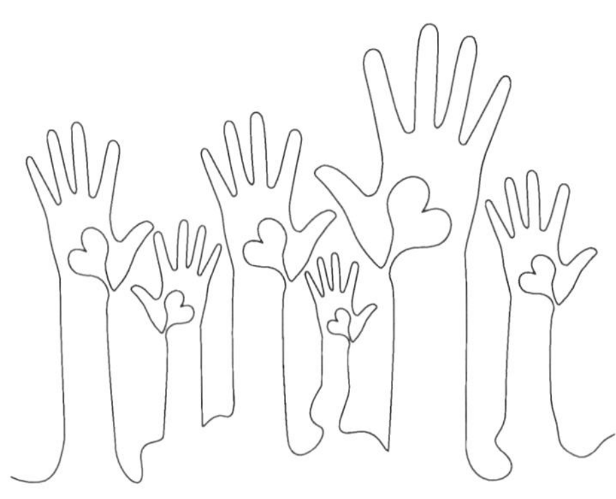

Joining an Online Community

Lymphie Strong is an online community for people with lymphatic diseases, including the Official Lymphie Strong Inspiration Group for Lymphedema on Facebook. Find more information at https://lymphiestrong.com/

The Lymphatic Education and Research Network (LE&RN) website has a lot of resources that can help you educate others on lymphedema https://lymphaticnetwork.org/

The Lymphie Strong list of Lymphedema Resources is at https://lymphiestrong.com/lymphedema-resources/

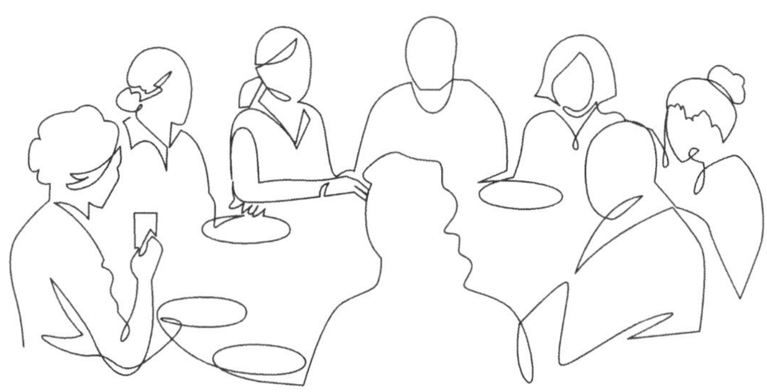

Working Together as Community

People with lymphedema also have difficulty with:

- Disinterested healthcare providers
- Government marginalization
- Social marginalization
- Lack of lymphedema research

- Lack of treatment resources
- Lack of insurance coverage for treatment and supplies
- Lack of choice in properly fitting clothes and shoes

Medical professionals need to join with people with lymphedema, their caregivers, family and friends to work together to solve these issues. We need:

- Lymphedema education and awareness for healthcare providers, members of the government, and the general public
- Programs that encourage people with lymphedema to be active members of their community
- Increased research, treatment resources, and insurance coverage
- Inclusive sizing in clothes and shoes

Let us know what else we need to work on here:

In the USA, we have just seen what the power of medical professionals and people with lymphedema can do when we join together. The Lymphedema Treatment Act was passed in 2022 after years of organized lobbying efforts. Learn more at: https://lymphedematreatmentact.org/

The National Lymphedema Network is a nonprofit that provides education and guidance regarding lymphedema management to patients, healthcare professionals, and the general public. Their website has resources you can use to inform healthcare professionals about lymphedema. Find out more at: https://lymphnet.org/

The Lymphatic Education and Research Network (LE&RN) is a nonprofit dedicated to education, research, and advocacy to improve the lives of those affected by lymphedema and lymphatic diseases including efforts to secure ongoing Congressional and National Institutes of Health (NIH) support for lymphatic research and lymphatic diseases. If you would like to get involved and connect with people affected by lymphedema and lymphatic diseases in your community, join your local LE&RN chapter. Find your local LE&RN chapter here: https://lymphaticnetwork.org/chapter-page

Conclusion

We looked at research and resources for working together as a community to advocate for the reduction of many of the situations which cause stress to people with lymphedema. Building a community reduces social isolation and working together as a community can empower us to advocate for lymphedema education and awareness as well as research, treatment resources and insurance coverage.

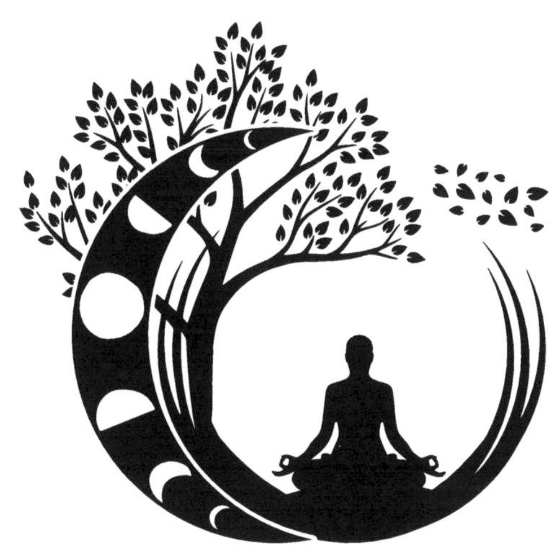

CHAPTER 9

FINAL THOUGHTS

I have shared a LOT of information! Let's begin this chapter with an opportunity for reflection.

Take time to be in a comfortable position and become aware of your body. Ask yourself these questions:

- What were your goals for reading this book?
- What did you read that has inspired you to learn more?
- What have you learned that will help you reduce stress levels?

- Which self-care practices really resonated with you?
- How will you bring what you have learned into your self-care practice and relationships with loved ones?

If you like journaling, I invite you to journal about these questions.

____

____

____

My goal was to share the importance of:

- Understanding the WHY behind self-care that lymphedema therapists recommend for our clients
- Encouraging people with lymphedema to appreciate their own voice of lived experience and try mindful interventions that have been shown to reduce stress

Our communities need:

- More public conversations around the negative effects of toxic stress, and about opportunities for self-care
- More access to physical and mental health resources
- More access to green spaces

- More opportunities for community engagement
- More health experts that can effectively spread awareness about lymphedema as well as stress reduction practices
- More research, treatment resources, and insurance coverage for lymphedema
- More inclusive sizing in clothes and shoes

This mission can only be accomplished through connecting with others and working together as a community where all voices are heard and honored. As Brene Brown says, changing or limiting ourselves to 'fit in' is the opposite of truly belonging.

People living with lymphedema will not benefit from a cookie-cutter approach of quick fixes that dismiss their lived experiences and need for safety and trust. I hope this book has increased awareness of the effects of stress on the mind and body and piqued interest in trying mindful interventions to reduce the negative effects of stress on health and wellbeing.

Thanks for taking the time to read this book. Connect with me on Instagram @StressReductionForLymphedema with any questions.

Two-week gratitude journal

Here is the protocol from researchers at the University of California, San Diego in the USA:

- Each day, record three to five things for which we are grateful
- Take time to remember our day and focus on everything that is a source of gratitude
- Personalize the list to our own experience
- Search for the little differences that happen every day, not just the big stuff

(Redwine et al., 2016)

Tips for keeping a gratitude journal

- Be specific: focus on the details of why and how the things in our life inspire gratitude
- Go in depth: spend a little time focusing on each item in the day's journal entry
- Focus on people as well as things: remember to also focus on people for whom we are grateful
- Keep it simple: we don't need a fancy journal or a timer to start practicing gratitude journaling
- Make it a habit: set aside a time and place to write in the journal if it's proving hard to adopt as a habit
- Don't make it a source of guilt: feeling gratitude shouldn't feel forced or make us feel guilty or ashamed. Some of us were embarrassed by loved ones and called "ungrateful" when we tried to advocate for our needs. Gratitude shouldn't feel manipulative

Questions at the beginning:

How strongly do you agree with the following statements? Rate agreement from 1 to 5 with 1 being "nope, not at all" and 5 being "absolutely agree."

- It's easy to find things to be grateful for throughout the day ___
- I have many things to be grateful for in the world ___
- I am grateful for the events and people in my life, both past and present ___

Day ____ Date ___________

Day ____ Date ___________

Day ____ Date ___________

Day ____ Date __________

Day ____ Date __________

Day ____ Date __________

Day ____ Date ___________

___

___

___

___

___

Day ____ Date ___________

___

___

___

___

___

Day ____ Date ___________

___

___

___

___

___

Day ____ Date __________

Day ____ Date __________

Day ____ Date __________

Day ____ Date ___________

____

____

____

____

____

Day ____ Date ___________

____

____

____

____

____

Questions at the End: How strongly do you agree with the following statements? Rate agreement from 1 to 5 with 1 being "nope, not at all" and 5 being "absolutely agree."

- It's easy to find things to be grateful for throughout the day ___
- I have many things to be grateful for in the world ___
- I am grateful for the events and people in my life, both past and present ___

Did your score change?

How do you feel after this practice?

____

____

____

RESOURCES

Abbasi B, Mirzakhany N, Angooti Oshnari L, Irani A, Hosseinzadeh S, Tabatabaei SM, Haghighat S. The effect of relaxation techniques on edema, anxiety and depression in post-mastectomy lymphedema patients undergoing comprehensive decongestive therapy: A clinical trial. PLoS One. 2018 Jan 5;13(1):e0190231. doi: 10.1371/journal.pone.0190231. PMID: 29304095; PMCID: PMC5755759. Retrieved from: https://www.ncbi.nlm.nih.gov/pmc/articles/PMC5755759/

Abebaw A, Atnafu A, Worku N, Hagos A. Health-related quality of life and associated factors among adult podoconiosis patients in Debre Elias district Northwest, Ethiopia. PLoS Negl Trop Dis. 2022 Sep 2;16(9):e0010673. doi: 10.1371/journal.pntd.0010673. PMID: 36054193; PMCID: PMC9477424. Retrieved from: https://www.ncbi.nlm.nih.gov/pmc/articles/PMC9477424/

Adhikari RK, Sherchand JB, Mishra SR, Ranabhat K, Pokharel A, Devkota P, Mishra D, Ghimire YC, Gelal K, Paudel R, Wagle RR. Health-seeking behaviors and self-care practices of people with filarial lymphoedema in Nepal: a qualitative study. J Trop Med. 2015;2015:260359. doi: 10.1155/2015/260359. Epub 2015 Jan 28. PMID: 25694785; PMCID: PMC4324917. Retrieved from: https://www.ncbi.nlm.nih.gov/pmc/articles/PMC4324917/

Aggithaya MG, Narahari SR, Ryan TJ. Yoga for correction of lymphedema's impairment of gait as an adjunct to lymphatic drainage: A pilot observational study. Int J Yoga. 2015 Jan;8(1):54-61. doi: 10.4103/0973-6131.146063. PMID: 25558134; PMCID: PMC4278136. Retrieved from: https://www.ncbi.nlm.nih.gov/pmc/articles/PMC4278136/

Albertson E, Neff, K., & Dill-Shackleford, K. (2014). Self-Compassion and Body Dissatisfaction in Women: A Randomized Controlled Trial of a Brief Meditation Intervention. Mindfulness. 6. . 10.1007/s12671-014-0277-3. Retrieved from: https://www.researchgate.net/publication/259941167_Self-Compassion_and_Body_Dissatisfaction_in_Women_A_Randomized_Controlled_Trial_of_a_Brief_Meditation_Intervention

Alem M, Gurgel MS. Acupuncture in the rehabilitation of women after breast cancer surgery. Acupunct Med 2008;26: 86-93. 23.

Allison PJ, Guichard C, Fung K, Gilain L. Dispositional optimism predicts survival status 1 year after diagnosis in head and neck cancer patients. J Clin Oncol. 2003 Feb 1;21(3):543-8. doi: 10.1200/JCO.2003.10.092. PMID: 12560447.

Amarasekera AT, Chang D. Buddhist meditation for vascular function: A narrative review. Integr Med Res. 2019 Dec;8(4):252-256. doi: 10.1016/j.imr.2019.11.002. Epub 2019 Nov 5. PMID: 31799114; PMCID: PMC6881634.

Retrieved from: https://www.ncbi.nlm.nih.gov/pmc/articles/PMC6881634/

Anderson, E. A., & Armer, J. M. (2021). Factors Impacting Management of Breast Cancer-Related Lymphedema (BCRL) in Hispanic/Latina Breast Cancer Survivors: A Literature Review. Hispanic Health Care International, 19(3), 190–202. doi:10.1177/1540415321990621 Retrieved from: https://www.ncbi.nlm.nih.gov/pmc/articles/PMC8353654/

Andersen TR. Regaining autonomy, competence, and relatedness: Experiences from two Shared Reading groups for people diagnosed with cancer. Front Psychol. 2022 Nov 1;13:1017166. doi: 10.3389/fpsyg.2022.1017166. PMID: 36389591; PMCID: PMC9665161. Retrieved from: https://www.ncbi.nlm.nih.gov/pmc/articles/PMC9665161/

Anjana K, Archana R, Mukkadan JK. Effect of om chanting and yoga nidra on blood pressure and lipid profile in hypertension - A randomized controlled trial. J Ayurveda Integr Med. 2022 Oct-Dec;13(4):100657. doi: 10.1016/j.jaim.2022.100657. Epub 2022 Nov 11. PMID: 36375220; PMCID: PMC9663516. Retrieved from: https://www.ncbi.nlm.nih.gov/pmc/articles/PMC9663516/

Arai YC, Sakakima Y, Kawanishi J, Nishihara M, Ito A, Tawada Y, Maruyama Y. Auricular acupuncture at the “shenmen” and “point zero” points induced parasympathetic activation. Evid Based

Complement Alternat Med. 2013;2013:945063. doi: 10.1155/2013/945063. Epub 2013 Jun 4. PMID: 23861718; PMCID: PMC3687596. Retrieved from: https://www.ncbi.nlm.nih.gov/pmc/articles/PMC3687596/

Arakaki X, Arechavala RJ, Choy EH, Bautista J, Bliss B, Molloy C, Wu DA, Shimojo S, Jiang Y, Kleinman MT, Kloner RA. The connection between heart rate variability (HRV), neurological health, and cognition: A literature review. Front Neurosci. 2023 Mar 1;17:1055445. doi: 10.3389/fnins.2023.1055445. PMID: 36937689; PMCID: PMC10014754. Retrieved from: https://www.ncbi.nlm.nih.gov/pmc/articles/PMC10014754/

Arinaga Y, Piller N, Sato F, Ishida T, Ohtake T, Kikuchi K, Sato-Tadano A, Tada H, Miyashita M. The 10-Min Holistic Self-Care for Patients with Breast Cancer-Related Lymphedema: Pilot Randomized Controlled Study. Tohoku J Exp Med. 2019 Feb;247(2):139-147. doi: 10.1620/tjem.247.139. PMID: 30799328. Retrieved from: https://www.jstage.jst.go.jp/article/tjem/247/2/247_139/_html/-char/en

Azam MA, Katz J, Fashler SR, Changoor T, Azargive S, Ritvo P. Heart rate variability is enhanced in controls but not maladaptive perfectionists during brief mindfulness meditation following stress-induction: A stratified-randomized trial. Int J Psychophysiol. 2015 Oct;98(1):27-34. doi: 10.1016/j.ijpsycho.2015.06.005. Epub 2015 Jun 25. PMID: 26116778. Retrieved from: https://core.ac.uk/download/pdf/77105399.pdf

Badger TA, Segrin C, Sikorskii A, Pasvogel A, Weihs K, Lopez AM, & Chalasani P (2020). Randomized controlled trial of supportive care interventions to manage psychological distress and symptoms in Latinas with breast cancer and their informal caregivers. *Psychology & Health*, 35(1), 87–106. 10.1080/08870446.2019.1626395 Retrieved from: https://repository.arizona.edu/bitstream/handle/10150/633364/RCT%20Psychological%20Distress%20and%20Symptoms%20in%20Latinas_Final_revised2019depository.pdf;jsessionid=F4DFD89396441D07B1C8851BF9845951?sequence=1

Bąk-Sosnowska M, Gruszczyńska M, Wyszomirska J, Daniel-Sielańczyk A. The Influence of Selected Psychological Factors on Medication Adherence in Patients with Chronic Diseases. Healthcare (Basel). 2022 Feb 24;10(3):426. doi: 10.3390/healthcare10030426. PMID: 35326906; PMCID: PMC8955226. Retrieved from: https://www.ncbi.nlm.nih.gov/pmc/articles/PMC8955226/

Balasubramanian S, Janech MG, Warren GW. Alterations in Salivary Proteome following Single Twenty-Minute Session of Yogic Breathing. Evid Based Complement Alternat Med. 2015;2015:376029. doi: 10.1155/2015/376029. Epub 2015 Mar 19. PMID: 25873979; PMCID: PMC4383272. Retrieved from: https://www.ncbi.nlm.nih.gov/pmc/articles/PMC4383272/

Balban MY, Neri E, Kogon MM, Weed L, Nouriani B, Jo B, Holl G, Zeitzer JM, Spiegel D, Huberman AD. Brief structured respiration practices enhance mood and reduce physiological arousal. Cell Rep Med. 2023 Jan 17;4(1):100895. doi: 10.1016/j.xcrm.2022.100895. Epub 2023 Jan 10. PMID: 36630953; PMCID: PMC9873947. Retrieved from: https://www.ncbi.nlm.nih.gov/pmc/articles/PMC9873947/

Basha, M.A., Aboelnour, N.H., Alsharidah, A.S. et al. Effect of exercise mode on physical function and quality of life in breast cancer–related lymphedema: a randomized trial. *Support Care Cancer* 30, 2101–2110 (2022). https://doi.org/10.1007/s00520-021-06559-1

Beecher ME, Eggett D, Erekson D, Rees LB, Bingham J, Klundt J, Bailey RJ, Ripplinger C, Kirchhoefer J, Gibson R, Griner D, Cox JC, Boardman RD. Sunshine on my shoulders: Weather, pollution, and emotional distress. J Affect Disord. 2016 Nov 15;205:234-238. doi: 10.1016/j.jad.2016.07.021. Epub 2016 Jul 16. PMID: 27449556.

https://www.sciencedirect.com/science/article/abs/pii/S0165032716306553

Begoglu FA, Akpinar P, Ozkan FU, Ozturk G, Aktas I. Health status, coronaphobia, quality of life, anxiety and depression in patients with lymphedema during COVID-19 pandemic. Lymphology. 2022;55(1):21-32. PMID: 35896112. Retrieved from: https://journals.librarypublishing.arizona.edu/lymph/article/id/5141/download/pdf/

Behman, P. J., Rash, J. A., Bagshawe, M., & Giesbrecht, J. (2018). Short-term autonomic nervous system and experiential responses during a labyrinth walk. *Cogent Psychology, 5*(1). Retrieved from: https://www.tandfonline.com/doi/full/10.1080/23311908.2018.1495036?src=recsys

Bennett MP, Lengacher C. Humor and Laughter May Influence Health: III. Laughter and Health Outcomes. Evid Based Complement Alternat Med. 2008 Mar;5(1):37-40. doi: 10.1093/ecam/nem041. PMID: 18317546; PMCID: PMC2249748. Retrieved from: https://www.ncbi.nlm.nih.gov/pmc/articles/PMC2249748/pdf/nem041.pdf

Bergmann A, Baiocchi JMT, de Andrade MFC. Conservative treatment of lymphedema: the state of the art. J Vasc Bras. 2021 Oct 11;20:e20200091. doi: 10.1590/1677-5449.200091. PMID: 34777487; PMCID: PMC8565523. Retrieved from: https://www.ncbi.nlm.nih.gov/pmc/articles/PMC8565523/

Bernardi L, Sleight P, Bandinelli G, Cencetti S, Fattorini L, Wdowczyc-Szulc J, Lagi A. Effect of rosary prayer and yoga mantras on autonomic cardiovascular rhythms: comparative study. BMJ. 2001 Dec 22-29;323(7327):1446-9. doi: 10.1136/bmj.323.7327.1446. PMID: 11751348; PMCID: PMC61046. Retrieved from: https://thaicam.go.th/wp-content/uploads/2019/06/148-1.pdf

Beukeboom, C. J., Langeveld, D., & Tanja-Dijkstra, K. (2012). Stress-reducing effects of real and artificial nature in a hospital waiting room. *Journal of Alternative Complementary Medicine, 18*(4):329-33. Retrieved from: https://core.ac.uk/reader/15476039?utm_source=linkout

Bock K, Ludwig R, Vaduvathiriyan P, LeSuer L, Siengsukon C. Sleep disturbance in cancer survivors with lymphedema: a scoping review. Support Care Cancer. 2022 Nov;30(11):9647-9657. doi: 10.1007/s00520-022-07378-8. Epub 2022 Oct 6. PMID: 36201052.

Bogan LK, Powell JM, Dudgeon BJ. Experiences of living with non-cancer-related lymphedema: implications for clinical practice. Qual Health Res. 2007 Feb;17(2):213-24. doi: 10.1177/1049732306297660. PMID: 17220392.

Bowman C, Oberoi D, Radke L, Francis GJ, Carlson LE. Living with leg lymphedema: developing a novel model of quality lymphedema care for cancer survivors. J Cancer Surviv. 2021 Feb;15(1):140-150. doi: 10.1007/s11764-020-00919-2. Epub 2020 Jul 26. PMID: 32712757; PMCID: PMC7822774. Retrieved from: https://www.ncbi.nlm.nih.gov/pmc/articles/PMC7822774/

Buki, L. P., Rivera-Ramos, Z. A., Kanagui-Muñoz, M., Heppner, P. P., Ojeda, L., Lehardy, E. N., & Weiterschan, K. A. (2021). "I never heard anything about it": Knowledge and psychosocial needs of Latina breast cancer survivors with lymphedema. *Women's Health, 17*, 17455065211002488. Retrieved from: https://journals.sagepub.com/doi/pdf/10.1177/17455065211002488

Cavezzi A. Medicine and Phlebolymphology: Time to Change? J Clin Med. 2020 Dec 18;9(12):4091. doi: 10.3390/jcm9124091. PMID: 33353052; PMCID: PMC7766771. Retrieved from: https://www.ncbi.nlm.nih.gov/pmc/articles/PMC7766771/

Chaieb, L., Wilpert, E. C., Reber, T. P., & Fell, J. (2015). Auditory beat stimulation and its effects on cognition and mood States. *Front Psychiatry, 6*(70). Retrieved from: https://www.ncbi.nlm.nih.gov/pmc/articles/PMC4428073/

Chayadi E, Baes N, Kiropoulos L. The effects of mindfulness-based interventions on symptoms of depression, anxiety, and cancer-related fatigue in oncology patients: A systematic review and meta-analysis. PLoS One. 2022 Jul 14;17(7):e0269519. doi: 10.1371/journal.pone.0269519. PMID: 35834503; PMCID: PMC9282451. Retrieved from: https://www.ncbi.nlm.nih.gov/pmc/articles/PMC9282451/

Cooper-Stanton GR, Gale N, Sidhu M, Allen K. A qualitative systematic review and meta-aggregation of the experiences of men diagnosed with chronic lymphoedema. J Res Nurs. 2022 Dec;27(8):704-732. doi: 10.1177/17449871221088791. Epub 2022 Sep 20. PMID: 36530746; PMCID: PMC9755568. Retrieved from: https://www.ncbi.nlm.nih.gov/pmc/articles/PMC9755568/

Cross RL, White J, Engelsher J, O'Connor SS. Implementation of Rocking Chair Therapy for Veterans in Residential Substance Use Disorder Treatment [Formula: see text]. J Am Psychiatr Nurses Assoc. 2018 May/Jun;24(3):190-198. doi: 10.1177/1078390317746726. Epub 2017 Dec 9. PMID: 29224460.

Davies C, Levenhagen K, Ryans K, Perdomo M, Gilchrist L. Interventions for Breast Cancer-Related Lymphedema: Clinical Practice Guideline From the Academy of Oncologic Physical Therapy of APTA. Phys Ther. 2020 Jul 19;100(7):1163-1179. doi: 10.1093/ptj/pzaa087. PMID: 32589208; PMCID: PMC7412854. Retrieved from: https://www.ncbi.nlm.nih.gov/pmc/articles/PMC7412854/

Davies EA. Why we need more poetry in palliative care. BMJ Support Palliat Care. 2018 Sep;8(3):266-270. doi: 10.1136/bmjspcare-2017-001477. Epub 2018 Mar 23. PMID: 29574424; PMCID: PMC6104682. Retrieved from: https://www.ncbi.nlm.nih.gov/pmc/articles/PMC6104682/

Davis, D. W. (2021). A literature review on the physiological and psychological effects of labyrinth walking. *Int J Yogic Hum Mov Sports Sci*, *6*(1), 167-175. Retrieved from: https://www.theyogicjournal.com/pdf/2021/vol6issue1/PartC/6-1-61-305.pdf

Delamerced, A., Panicker, C., Monteiro, K., & Chung, E. Y. (2021). Effects of a poetry intervention on emotional wellbeing in hospitalized pediatric patients. *Hospital Pediatrics, 11*(3), 263-269. Retrieved from: https://pubmed.ncbi.nlm.nih.gov/33622762/

Dominick SA, Natarajan L, Pierce JP, Madanat H, Madlensky L. The psychosocial impact of lymphedema-related distress among breast cancer survivors in the WHEL Study. Psychooncology. 2014 Sep;23(9):1049-56. doi: 10.1002/pon.3510. Epub 2014 Feb 26. PMID: 24615880; PMCID: PMC4145047. Retrieved from: https://www.ncbi.nlm.nih.gov/pmc/articles/PMC4145047/

Douglass, Jan & Immink, Maarten & Piller, Neil & Ullah, Shahid. (2012). Yoga for women with breast cancer-related lymphoedema: A preliminary 6-month study. Journal of Lymphoedema. 7. 30-38. Retrieved from: https://www.researchgate.net/publication/257748548_Yoga_for_women_with_breast_cancer-related_lymphoedema_A_preliminary_6-month_study

Douglass J, Mableson HE, Martindale S, Kelly-Hope LA. An Enhanced Self-Care Protocol for People Affected by Moderate to Severe Lymphedema. Methods Protoc. 2019 Sep 4;2(3):77. doi: 10.3390/mps2030077. PMID: 31487887; PMCID: PMC6789820. Retrieved from: https://www.ncbi.nlm.nih.gov/pmc/articles/PMC6789820/

B Douglass J, Hailekiros F, Martindale S, Mableson H, Seife F, Bishaw T, Nigussie M, Meribo K, Tamiru M, Agidew G, Kim S, Betts H, Taylor M, Kelly-Hope L. Addition of Lymphatic Stimulating Self-Care Practices Reduces Acute Attacks among People Affected by Moderate and Severe Lower-Limb Lymphedema in Ethiopia, a Cluster Randomized Controlled Trial. J Clin Med. 2020 Dec 17;9(12):4077. doi: 10.3390/jcm9124077.

PMID: 33348721; PMCID: PMC7766500. Retrieved from: https://www.ncbi.nlm.nih.gov/pmc/articles/PMC7766500/

Douglass J, Mableson H, Martindale S, Jhara ST, Karim MJ, Rahman MM, Kawsar AA, Khair A, Mahmood AS, Rahman AF, Chowdhury SM, Kim S, Betts H, Taylor M, Kelly-Hope L. Effect of an Enhanced Self-Care Protocol on Lymphedema Status among People Affected by Moderate to Severe Lower-Limb Lymphedema in Bangladesh, a Cluster Randomized Controlled Trial. J Clin Med. 2020 Jul 30;9(8):2444. doi: 10.3390/jcm9082444. PMID: 32751676; PMCID: PMC7464742. Retrieved from: https://www.ncbi.nlm.nih.gov/pmc/articles/PMC7464742/

Dragoş D, Tănăsescu MD. The effect of stress on the defense systems. J Med Life. 2010 Jan-Mar;3(1):10-8. PMID: 20302192; PMCID: PMC3019042. Retrieved from: https://pubmed.ncbi.nlm.nih.gov/20302192/

Dreisoerner, A., Junker, N.M., Schlotz, W., Heimrich, J., Bloemeke, S., Ditzen, B., & van Dick, R. (2021). Self-soothing touch and being hugged reduce cortisol responses to stress: A randomized controlled trial on stress, physical touch, and social identity. *Comprehensive Psychoneuroendocrinology.*

Retrieved from: https://www.sciencedirect.com/science/article/pii/S2666497621000655?via%3Dihub&ck_subscriber_id=157723643

Duhon BH, Phan TT, Taylor SL, Crescenzi RL, Rutkowski JM. Current Mechanistic Understandings of Lymphedema and Lipedema: Tales of Fluid, Fat, and Fibrosis. Int J Mol Sci. 2022 Jun 14;23(12):6621. doi: 10.3390/ijms23126621. PMID: 35743063; PMCID: PMC9223758. Retrieved from: https://www.ncbi.nlm.nih.gov/pmc/articles/PMC9223758/

Eid, C. M., Hamilton, C., Greer, J. M. H. (2022). Untangling the tingle: Investigating the association between the autonomous sensory meridian response (ASMR), neuroticism, and trait & state anxiety. *PLoS One,17*(2), e0262668. Retrieved from: https://www.ncbi.nlm.nih.gov/pmc/articles/PMC8809551/

Ein, N, Li, L., & Vickers, K. The effect of pet therapy on the physiological and subjective stress response: A meta-analysis. *Stress Health, 34*(4), 477-489. Retrieved from: https://pubmed.ncbi.nlm.nih.gov/29882342/

Fancourt D, Williamon A, Carvalho LA, Steptoe A, Dow R, Lewis I. Singing modulates mood, stress, cortisol, cytokine and neuropeptide activity in cancer patients and carers. Ecancermedicalscience. 2016 Apr 5;10:631. doi: 10.3332/ecancer.2016.631. PMID: 27170831; PMCID: PMC4854222. Retrieved from: https://www.ncbi.nlm.nih.gov/pmc/articles/PMC4854222/

Farley H. Promoting self-efficacy in patients with chronic disease beyond traditional education: A literature review. Nurs Open. 2019 Oct 20;7(1):30-41. doi: 10.1002/

nop2.382. PMID: 31871689; PMCID: PMC6917929. Retrieved from: https://www.ncbi.nlm.nih.gov/pmc/articles/PMC6917929/

Farrar, A. J., & Farrar, F. C. (2020). Clinical aromatherapy. *Nurse Clin North Am, 55*(4), 489-504. Retrieved from: https://www.ncbi.nlm.nih.gov/pmc/articles/PMC7520654/

Finnane A, Liu Y, Battistutta D, Janda M, Hayes SC. Lymphedema after breast or gynecological cancer: use and effectiveness of mainstream and complementary therapies. J Altern Complement Med. 2011 Sep;17(9):867-9. doi: 10.1089/acm.2010.0456. PMID: 21875352. Retrieved from: https://eprints.qut.edu.au/46303/1/46303.pdf

Fisher MI, Donahoe-Fillmore B, Leach L, O'Malley C, Paeplow C, Prescott T, Merriman H. Effects of yoga on arm volume among women with breast cancer related lymphedema: A pilot study. J Bodyw Mov Ther. 2014 Oct;18(4):559-65. doi: 10.1016/j.jbmt.2014.02.006. Epub 2014 Mar 1. PMID: 25440207. Retrieved from: https://ecommons.udayton.edu/cgi/viewcontent.cgi?article=1017&context=dpt_fac_pub

Fong SS, Ng SS, Luk WS, Chung JW, Ho JS, Ying M, Ma AW. Effects of qigong exercise on upper limb lymphedema and blood flow in survivors of breast cancer: a pilot study. Integr Cancer Ther. 2014 Jan;13(1):54-61. doi: 10.1177/1534735413490797. Epub

2013 Jun 7. PMID: 23749481. Retrieved from: https://journals.sagepub.com/doi/10.1177/1534735413490797

Frid M, Strang P, Friedrichsen MJ, Johansson K. Lower Limb Lymphedema: Experiences and Perceptions of Cancer Patients in the Late Palliative Stage. *Journal of Palliative Care*. 2006;22(1):5-11. doi:10.1177/082585970602200102

Frostadottir, A. D., & Dorjee, D. (2019). Effects of mindfulness-based cognitive therapy (MBCT) and compassion-focused therapy (CFT) on symptom change, mindfulness, self-compassion, and rumination in clients with depression, anxiety, and stress. *Frontiers in Psychology*, *10*, 1099. Retrieved from: https://www.ncbi.nlm.nih.gov/pmc/articles/PMC6534108/

Fu MR, Ridner SH, Hu SH, Stewart BR, Cormier JN, Armer JM. Psychosocial impact of lymphedema: a systematic review of literature from 2004 to 2011. Psychooncology. 2013 Jul;22(7):1466-84. doi: 10.1002/pon.3201. Epub 2012 Oct 9. PMID: 23044512; PMCID: PMC4153404. Retrieved from: https://www.ncbi.nlm.nih.gov/pmc/articles/PMC4153404/

Fu MR, McTernan ML, Qiu JM, Ko E, Yazicioglu S, Axelrod D, Guth A, Fan Z, Sang A, Miaskowski C, Wang Y. The Effects of Kinect-Enhanced Lymphatic Exercise Intervention on Lymphatic Pain, Swelling, and Lymph Fluid Level. Integr Cancer Ther. 2021 Jan-Dec;20:15347354211026757. doi:

10.1177/15347354211026757. PMID: 34160294; PMCID: PMC8226364. Retrieved from: https://www.ncbi.nlm.nih.gov/pmc/articles/PMC8226364/

Fu MR, Axelrod D, Guth AA, Scagliola J, Rampertaap K, El-Shammaa N, Qiu JM, McTernan ML, Frye L, Park CS, Yu G, Tilley C, Wang Y

A Web- and Mobile-Based Intervention for Women Treated for Breast Cancer to Manage Chronic Pain and Symptoms Related to Lymphedema: Results of a Randomized Clinical Trial

JMIR Cancer 2022;8(1):e29485 doi: 10.2196/29485 Retrieved from: https://cancer.jmir.org/2022/1/e29485/

Gandhi A, Xu T, DeSnyder SM, Smith GL, Lin R, Barcenas CH, Stauder MC, Hoffman KE, Strom EA, Ferguson S, Smith BD, Woodward WA, Perkins GH, Mitchell MP, Garner D, Goodman CR, Aldrich M, Travis M, Lilly S, Bedrosian I, Shaitelman SF. Prospective, early longitudinal assessment of lymphedema-related quality of life among patients with locally advanced breast cancer: The foundation for building a patient-centered screening program. Breast. 2023 Feb 24;68:205-215. doi: 10.1016/j.breast.2023.02.011. Epub ahead of print. PMID: 36863241; PMCID: PMC9996356. Retrieved from: https://www.ncbi.nlm.nih.gov/pmc/articles/PMC9996356/

Gencay Can A, Can SS, Ekşioğlu E, Çakcı FA. Is kinesiophobia associated with lymphedema, upper extremity function, and psychological morbidity in breast cancer survivors? Turk J Phys Med Rehabil. 2018 Aug 12;65(2):139-146. doi: 10.5606/tftrd.2019.2585. PMID: 31453554; PMCID: PMC6706825. Retrieved from: https://www.ncbi.nlm.nih.gov/pmc/articles/PMC6706825/

Germer, C. K., & Neff, K. (2019). *Teaching the mindful self-compassion program: A guide for professionals*. The Guilford Press.

Gianesini S, Tessari M, Baccaglieri P, Malagoni AM, Menegatti E, Occhionorelli S, Basaglia N, Zamboni P. A specifically designed aquatic exercise protocol to reduce chronic lower limb edema. Phlebology. 2017 Oct;32(9):594-600. doi: 10.1177/0268355516673539. Epub 2016 Oct 18. PMID: 27756859. Retrieved from: https://iris.unife.it/bitstream/11392/2354652/4/0268355516673539.pdf

Gonzalez BD, Eisel SL, Qin B, Llanos AAM, Savard J, Hoogland AI, Jim H, Lin Y, Demissie K, Hong CC, Bandera EV. Prevalence, risk factors, and trajectories of sleep disturbance in a cohort of African-American breast cancer survivors. Support Care Cancer. 2021 May;29(5):2761-2770. doi: 10.1007/s00520-020-05786-2. Epub 2020 Sep 29. PMID: 32995999; PMCID: PMC7981240. Retrieved from: https://www.ncbi.nlm.nih.gov/pmc/articles/PMC7981240/

Gore, M. M. (2005). *Anatomy and Physiology of Yogic Practices*. New Age Books.

Graff, V., Cai, L., Badiola, I., & Elkassabany, N. M. (2018). Music versus midazolam during preoperative nerve block placements: A prospective randomized controlled study. *Reg Anesth Pain Med*icine. Retrieved from: https://sbgg.org.br/wp-content/uploads/2019/07/1563905859_1_Music_versus_midazolam.pdf

Greenlee H, DuPont-Reyes MJ, Balneaves LG, Carlson LE, Cohen MR, Deng G, Johnson JA, Mumber M, Seely D, Zick SM, Boyce LM, Tripathy D. Clinical practice guidelines on the evidence-based use of integrative therapies during and after breast cancer treatment. CA Cancer J Clin. 2017 May 6;67(3):194-232. doi: 10.3322/caac.21397. Epub 2017 Apr 24. PMID: 28436999; PMCID: PMC5892208. Retrieved from: https://www.ncbi.nlm.nih.gov/pmc/articles/PMC5892208/

Hamilton JB, Worthy VC, Kurtz MJ, Cudjoe J, Johnstone PA. Using Religious Songs as an Integrative and Complementary Therapy for the Management of Psychological Symptoms Among African American Cancer Survivors. Cancer Nurs. 2016 Nov/Dec;39(6):488-494. doi: 10.1097/NCC.0000000000000335. PMID: 26859281.

Hansen MM, Jones R, Tocchini K. Shinrin-Yoku (Forest Bathing) and Nature Therapy: A State-of-the-Art Review. Int J Environ Res Public Health. 2017 Jul 28;14(8):851. doi: 10.3390/ijerph14080851. PMID: 28788101; PMCID: PMC5580555. Retrieved from: https://www.ncbi.nlm.nih.gov/pmc/articles/PMC5580555/

Haynes-Maslow, L., Allicock, M., & Johnson, L.-S. (2015). *Cancer Support Needs for African American Breast Cancer Survivors and Caregivers. Journal of Cancer Education, 31(1), 166–171.* doi:10.1007/s13187-015-0832-1 Retrieved from: https://sci-hub.ru/10.1007/s13187-015-0832-1

He L, Qu H, Wu Q, Song Y. Lymphedema in survivors of breast cancer. Oncol Lett. 2020 Mar;19(3):2085-2096. doi: 10.3892/ol.2020.11307. Epub 2020 Jan 16. PMID: 32194706; PMCID: PMC7039097. Retrieved from: https://www.ncbi.nlm.nih.gov/pmc/articles/PMC7039097/

Heart Rate Variability (2021, September 1). Retrieved from: https://my.clevelandclinic.org/health/symptoms/21773-heart-rate-variability-hrv

Henderson, P. G., Rosen, D. H., & Mascaro, N. (2007). Empirical study on the healing nature of mandalas. *Psychology of Aesthetics, Creativity, and the Arts, 1*, 148-154.

Hotho G, von Bonin D, Krüerke D, Wolf U, Cysarz D. Unexpected Cardiovascular Oscillations at 0.1 Hz During Slow Speech Guided Breathing (OM Chanting) at 0.05 Hz. Front Physiol. 2022 May 10;13:875583. doi: 10.3389/fphys.2022.875583. PMID: 35620613; PMCID: PMC9127736. Retrieved from: https://www.ncbi.nlm.nih.gov/pmc/articles/PMC9127736/

Inoue K, Maruoka H. Effects of simplified lymph drainage on the body: in females with menopausal disorder. J

Phys Ther Sci. 2017 Jan;29(1):115-118. doi: 10.1589/jpts.29.115. Epub 2017 Jan 30. PMID: 28210055; PMCID: PMC5300821.

Retrieved from: https://www.ncbi.nlm.nih.gov/pmc/articles/PMC5300821

Involving Patients in Care: Debridement Considerations. (2022, April 30). Retrieved from: https://www.woundsource.com/blog/involving-patients-in-care-debridement-considerations

Jin H, Xiang Y, Feng Y, Zhang Y, Liu S, Ruan S, Zhou H. Effectiveness and Safety of Acupuncture Moxibustion Therapy Used in Breast Cancer-Related Lymphedema: A Systematic Review and Meta-Analysis. Evid Based Complement Alternat Med. 2020 May 11;2020:3237451. doi: 10.1155/2020/3237451. PMID: 32454855; PMCID: PMC7240793. Retrieved from: https://www.ncbi.nlm.nih.gov/pmc/articles/PMC7240793/

Kahana-Zweig R, Geva-Sagiv M, Weissbrod A, Secundo L, Soroker N, Sobel N. Measuring and Characterizing the Human Nasal Cycle. PLoS One. 2016 Oct 6;11(10):e0162918. doi: 10.1371/journal.pone.0162918. PMID: 27711189; PMCID: PMC5053491 Retrieved from: https://www.ncbi.nlm.nih.gov/pmc/articles/PMC5053491/

Kai S, Nagino K, Aoki T, Imura T, Kiyoshima K, Satake Y, Matsuura K, Mima K, Yasuoka S, Yabuuchi A. Cardiac Autonomic Nervous System Activity during

Slow Breathing in Supine Position. Rehabil Res Pract. 2021 Feb 27;2021:6619571. doi: 10.1155/2021/6619571. PMID: 33728068; PMCID: PMC7936890. Retrieved from: https://www.ncbi.nlm.nih.gov/pmc/articles/PMC7936890/

Kalemikerakis I, Evaggelakou A, Kavga A, Vastardi M, Konstantinidis T, Govina O. Diagnosis, treatment and quality of life in patients with cancer-related lymphedema. J BUON. 2021 Sep-Oct;26(5):1735-1741. PMID: 34761576. Retrieved from: https://www.jbuon.com/archive/26-5-1735.pdf

Keser I, Esmer M. Does Manual Lymphatic Drainage Have Any Effect on Pain Threshold and Tolerance of Different Body Parts? Lymphat Res Biol. 2019 Dec;17(6):651-654. doi: 10.1089/lrb.2019.0005. Epub 2019 Jul 19. PMID: 31329499. Retrieved from: https://www.researchgate.net/profile/Murat-Esmer/publication/334623092_Does_Manual_Lymphatic_Drainage_Have_Any_Effect_on_Pain_Threshold_and_Tolerance_of_Different_Body_Parts/links/5ea47f02299bf112560e6a64/Does-Manual-Lymphatic-Drainage-Have-Any-Effect-on-Pain-Threshold-and-Tolerance-of-Different-Body-Parts.pdf

Khodabakhshi-Koolaee, A., & Darestani-Farahani, F. (2020). Mandala Coloring as Jungian Art to Reduce Bullying and Increase Social Skills. Retrieved from: https://jccnc.iums.ac.ir/article-1-269-fa.pdf

Kiecolt-Glaser JK, Bennett JM, Andridge R, Peng J, Shapiro CL, Malarkey WB, Emery CF, Layman R, Mrozek EE, Glaser R. Yoga's impact on inflammation, mood, and fatigue in breast cancer survivors: a randomized controlled trial. J Clin Oncol. 2014 Apr 1;32(10):1040-9. doi: 10.1200/JCO.2013.51.8860. Epub 2014 Jan 27. PMID: 24470004; PMCID: PMC3965259. Retrieved from: https://www.ncbi.nlm.nih.gov/pmc/articles/PMC3965259/

Kim SJ, Kwon OY, Yi CH. Effects of manual lymph drainage on cardiac autonomic tone in healthy subjects. Int J Neurosci. 2009;119(8):1105-17. doi: 10.1080/00207450902834884. PMID: 19922342. Retrieved from: https://static1.squarespace.com/static/5c292c6025bf0234971b23f0/t/5d1692d29807aa0001595c05/1561760467430/MLD+and+cardiac+autonomic+tone+-+Kim+3.pdf

Kim SH, Schneider SM, Kravitz L, Mermier C, Burge MR. Mind-body practices for posttraumatic stress disorder. J Investig Med. 2013 Jun;61(5):827-34. doi: 10.2310/JIM.0b013e3182906862. PMID: 23609463; PMCID: PMC3668544. Retrieved from: https://www.ncbi.nlm.nih.gov/pmc/articles/PMC3668544/

Kim, S. (2014). Effects of Manual Lymph Drainage on the Activity of Sympathetic Nervous System, Anxiety, Pain, and Pressure Pain Threshold in Subjects with Psychological Stress. *The Journal of Korean Physical Therapy, 26*, 391-397.

https://koreascience.kr/article/JAKO201425257248775.pdf

Kim SH, Kim YH, Kim HJ. Laughter and Stress Relief in Cancer Patients: A Pilot Study. Evid Based Complement Alternat Med. 2015;2015:864739. doi: 10.1155/2015/864739. Epub 2015 May 24. PMID: 26064177; PMCID: PMC4439472. Retrieved from: https://www.ncbi.nlm.nih.gov/pmc/articles/PMC4439472/

Kim H, Newman MG. The paradox of relaxation training: Relaxation induced anxiety and mediation effects of negative contrast sensitivity in generalized anxiety disorder and major depressive disorder. J Affect Disord. 2019 Dec 1;259:271-278. doi: 10.1016/j.jad.2019.08.045. Epub 2019 Aug 19. PMID: 31450137; PMCID: PMC7288612. Retrieved from: https://www.ncbi.nlm.nih.gov/pmc/articles/PMC7288612/

Ko, M. (2021). The Effect of Manual Lymphatic Drainage on the Stress and Pain in Patient with Postoperative Breast Cancer. *Physical Therapy Rehabilitation Science*. Retrieved from: https://pdfs.semanticscholar.org/0a1f/308d03cfdafabb7db0ff7f4b20f32408a2f8.pdf?_gl=1*9rtovt*_ga*MTE0MjEzMzA3NS4xNjc2MjM3NzU4*_ga_H7P4ZT52H5*MTY3OTQ1OTM3NC41LjEuMTY3OTQ2MDQ3OC4wLjAuMA..

Kocjan J, Adamek M, Gzik-Zroska B, Czyżewski D, Rydel M. Network of breathing. Multifunctional role of the diaphragm: a review. Adv Respir Med. 2017;85(4):224-232. doi: 10.5603/ARM.2017.0037. PMID: 28871591. Retrieved from: https://journals.viamedica.pl/advances in respiratory medicine/article/view/ARM.2017.0037/41543

Kumar A, Kala N, Telles S. Cerebrovascular Dynamics Associated with Yoga Breathing and Breath Awareness. Int J Yoga. 2022 Jan-Apr;15(1):19-24. doi: 10.4103/ijoy.ijoy_179_21. Epub 2022 Mar 21. PMID: 35444370; PMCID: PMC9015084. Retrieved from: https://www.ncbi.nlm.nih.gov/pmc/articles/PMC9015084/

Kuppusamy M, Kamaldeen D, Pitani R, Amaldas J, Shanmugam P. Effects of *Bhramari Pranayama* on health - A systematic review. J Tradit Complement Med. 2017 Mar 18;8(1):11-16. doi: 10.1016/j.jtcme.2017.02.003. PMID: 29321984; PMCID: PMC5755957. Retrieved: https://www.ncbi.nlm.nih.gov/pmc/articles/PMC5755957/pdf/main.pdf

Larsson SC, Lee WH, Kar S, Burgess S, Allara E. Assessing the role of cortisol in cancer: a wide-ranged Mendelian randomisation study. Br J Cancer. 2021 Sep;125(7):1025-1029. doi: 10.1038/s41416-021-01505-8. Epub 2021 Jul 27. PMID: 34316022; PMCID: PMC8476513. Retrieved from: https://www.ncbi.nlm.nih.gov/pmc/articles/PMC8476513/

Le CP, Sloan EK. Stress-driven lymphatic dissemination: An unanticipated consequence of communication between the sympathetic nervous system and lymphatic vasculature. Mol Cell Oncol. 2016 May 31;3(4):e1177674. doi: 10.1080/23723556.2016.1177674. PMID: 27652324; PMCID: PMC4972108. Retrieved from: https://www.ncbi.nlm.nih.gov/pmc/articles/PMC4972108/

Lemanne, D., & Maizes, V. (2018). Advising Women Undergoing Treatment for Breast Cancer: A Narrative Review. *Journal of alternative and complementary medicine, 24 9-10*, 902-909. Retrieved from: https://sci-hub.ru/10.1089/acm.2018.0150

LEVI L. THE URINARY OUTPUT OF ADRENALIN AND NORADRENALIN DURING PLEASANT AND UNPLEASANT EMOTIONAL STATES. A PRELIMINARY REPORT. Psychosom Med. 1965 Jan-Feb;27:80-5. doi: 10.1097/00006842-196501000-00009. PMID: 14258699. Retrieved from: https://psycnet.apa.org/record/1965-11651-001

Liljencrantz J, Strigo I, Ellingsen DM, Krämer HH, Lundblad LC, Nagi SS, Leknes S, Olausson H. Slow brushing reduces heat pain in humans. Eur J Pain. 2017 Aug;21(7):1173-1185. doi: 10.1002/ejp.1018. Epub 2017 Mar 6. PMID: 28263013.

Lin Y, Fisher ME, Roberts SM, Moser JS. Deconstructing the Emotion Regulatory Properties of Mindfulness: An Electrophysiological Investigation. Front Hum Neurosci. 2016 Sep 7;10:451. doi: 10.3389/fnhum.2016.00451. PMID: 27656139; PMCID: PMC5013076. Retrieved from: https://www.ncbi.nlm.nih.gov/pmc/articles/PMC5013076/

Lizarraga-Valderrama LR. Effects of essential oils on central nervous system: Focus on mental health. Phytother Res. 2021 Feb;35(2):657-679. doi: 10.1002/ptr.6854. Epub 2020 Aug 29. PMID: 32860651. Retrieved from: https://onlinelibrary.wiley.com/doi/pdfdirect/10.1002/ptr.6854

Lizier, D. S., Silva-Filho, R., Umada, J., Melo, R., & Neves, A. C. (2018). Effects of reflective labyrinth walking assessed using a questionnaire. *Medicines*, *5*(4), 111. Retrieved from: https://www.ncbi.nlm.nih.gov/pmc/articles/PMC6313772/

Loudon A, Barnett T, Piller N, Immink MA, Williams AD. Yoga management of breast cancer-related lymphoedema: a randomised controlled pilot-trial. BMC Complement Altern Med. 2014 Jul 1;14:214. doi: 10.1186/1472-6882-14-214. PMID: 24980836; PMCID: PMC4083036. Retrieved from: https://www.ncbi.nlm.nih.gov/pmc/articles/PMC4083036/pdf/1472-6882-14-214.pdf

Loudon A, Barnett T, Williams A. Yoga, breast cancer-related lymphoedema and well-being: A descriptive report of women's participation in a clinical trial. J Clin Nurs. 2017 Dec;26(23-24):4685-4695. doi: 10.1111/jocn.13819. Epub 2017 Jun 22. PMID: 28334470. Retrieved from: https://www.semanticscholar.org/

paper/Yoga%2C-breast-cancer%E2%80%90related-lymphoedema-and-A-of-in-Loudon-Barnett/048764952dd0dd1d3fb8d99aa35fac812c03d7c7

Luberto CM, McLeish AC, Kallen RW. Development and Initial Validation of the Relaxation Sensitivity Index. Int J Cogn Ther. 2021 Jun;14(2):320-340. doi: 10.1007/s41811-020-00086-3. Epub 2020 Sep 4. PMID: 34149986; PMCID: PMC8210687. Retrieved from: https://www.ncbi.nlm.nih.gov/pmc/articles/PMC8210687/

Lupis SB, Sabik NJ, Wolf JM. Role of shame and body esteem in cortisol stress responses. J Behav Med. 2016 Apr;39(2):262-75. doi: 10.1007/s10865-015-9695-5. Epub 2015 Nov 17. PMID: 26577952; PMCID: PMC5125296. Retrieved from: https://www.ncbi.nlm.nih.gov/pmc/articles/PMC5125296/

Lymphatic Education & Research Network. (2019, Dec. 3). Addressing the Emotional Stress of Living with a Chronic Disease - Leora Lowenthal, LICSW. [Video]. YouTube. https://youtu.be/PqOhac3SaTs

Ma X, Yue ZQ, Gong ZQ, Zhang H, Duan NY, Shi YT, Wei GX, Li YF. The Effect of Diaphragmatic Breathing on Attention, Negative Affect and Stress in Healthy Adults. Front Psychol. 2017 Jun 6;8:874. doi: 10.3389/fpsyg.2017.00874. PMID: 28626434; PMCID: PMC5455070. Retrieved from: https://www.researchgate.net/publication/317672754_The_Effect_

of Diaphragmatic Breathing on Attention Negative Affect and Stress in Healthy Adults

Maccarone MC, Venturini E, Menegatti E, Gianesini S, Masiero S. Water-based exercise for upper and lower limb lymphedema treatment. J Vasc Surg Venous Lymphat Disord. 2023 Jan;11(1):201-209. doi: 10.1016/j.jvsv.2022.08.002. Epub 2022 Aug 20. PMID: 35995327.

Martarelli D, Cocchioni M, Scuri S, Pompei P. Diaphragmatic breathing reduces exercise-induced oxidative stress. Evid Based Complement Alternat Med. 2011;2011:932430. doi: 10.1093/ecam/nep169. Epub 2011 Feb 10. PMID: 19875429; PMCID: PMC3139518. Retrieved from: https://www.ncbi.nlm.nih.gov/pmc/articles/PMC3139518/

McClure, M. K., McClure, R. J., Day, R., & Brufsky, A. M. (2010). Randomized controlled trial of the Breast Cancer Recovery Program for women with breast cancer–related lymphedema. *The American Journal of Occupational Therapy*, *64*(1), 59-72.

Meevissen YM, Peters ML, Alberts HJ. Become more optimistic by imagining a best possible self: effects of a two week intervention. J Behav Ther Exp Psychiatry. 2011 Sep;42(3):371-8. doi: 10.1016/j.jbtep.2011.02.012. Epub 2011 Mar 2. PMID: 21450262. Retrieved from: https://cris.maastrichtuniversity.nl/ws/portalfiles/portal/76692898/Peters 2011 Become more optimistic by imagining.pdf

Meier M, Wirz L, Dickinson P, Pruessner JC. Laughter yoga reduces the cortisol response to acute stress in healthy individuals. Stress. 2021 Jan;24(1):44-52. doi: 10.1080/10253890.2020.1766018. Epub 2020 May 26. PMID: 32393092. Retrieved from: https://kops.uni-konstanz.de/server/api/core/bitstreams/5d15a541-5da1-4162-a86a-7b7d42781c6a/content

Menziletoglu, D., Guler, A. Y., Cayır, T., & Isik, B. K. (2018). Binaural beats or 432 Hz music? Which method is more effective for reducing preoperative dental anxiety? *Med Oral Patol Oral Cir Bucal, 26*(1):e97-e101. Retrieved from: https://www.ncbi.nlm.nih.gov/pmc/articles/PMC7806348/

Mind and Body Practices (2017) Retrieved from: https://www.nccih.nih.gov/health/mind-and-body-practices

Mitten D, Overholt JR, Haynes FI, D'Amore CC, Ady JC. Hiking: A Low-Cost, Accessible Intervention to Promote Health Benefits. Am J Lifestyle Med. 2016 Jul 9;12(4):302-310. doi: 10.1177/1559827616658229. PMID: 32063815; PMCID: PMC6993091. Retrieved from: https://www.ncbi.nlm.nih.gov/pmc/articles/PMC6993091/

Morgan PA, Franks PJ, Moffatt CJ. Health-related quality of life with lymphoedema: a review of the literature. Int Wound J. 2005 Mar;2(1):47-62. doi: 10.1111/j.1742-4801.2005.00066.x. PMID: 16722853; PMCID:

PMC7951421. Retrieved from: https://www.ncbi.nlm.nih.gov/pmc/articles/PMC7951421/

Morishima T, Miyashiro I, Inoue N, Kitasaka M, Akazawa T, Higeno A, Idota A, Sato A, Ohira T, Sakon M, Matsuura N. Effects of laughter therapy on quality of life in patients with cancer: An open-label, randomized controlled trial. PLoS One. 2019 Jun 27;14(6):e0219065. doi: 10.1371/journal.pone.0219065. PMID: 31247017; PMCID: PMC6597115. Retrieved from: https://www.ncbi.nlm.nih.gov/pmc/articles/PMC6597115/pdf/pone.0219065.pdf

Moseley AL, Piller NB, Carati CJ. The effect of gentle arm exercise and deep breathing on secondary arm lymphedema. Lymphology. 2005 Sep;38(3):136-45. PMID: 16353491.

Retrieved from: https://www.researchgate.net/publication/7417505 The effect of gentle arm exercise and deep breathing on secondary arm lymphedema

Narahari SR, Ryan TJ, Mahadevan PE, Bose KS, Prasanna KS. Integrated management of filarial lymphedema for rural communities. Lymphology. 2007 Mar;40(1):3-13. PMID: 17539459.

Narahari SR, Aggithaya MG, Thernoe L, Bose KS, Ryan TJ. Yoga protocol for treatment of breast cancer-related lymphedema. Int J Yoga. 2016 Jul-Dec;9(2):145-55. doi: 10.4103/0973-6131.183713. PMID: 27512322; PMCID:

PMC4959325. Retrieved from: https://www.ncbi.nlm.nih.gov/pmc/articles/PMC4959325/

Narahari, S. R.. Integrative medicine for global health program of morbidity management and disability prevention of lymphedema. International Journal of Ayurveda Research 3(2):p 80-83, Jul–Dec 2022. | DOI: 10.4103/ijar.ijar_30_22 Retrieved from: https://journals.lww.com/ijar/Fulltext/2022/07000/Integrative_medicine_for_global_health_program_of.2.aspx

Neff, K. (n.d.) Why We Need to Have Compassion for Our Inner Critic. Retrieved from: https://self-compassion.org/why-we-need-to-have-compassion-for-our-inner-critic/

Obrero-Gaitán E, Cortés-Pérez I, Calet-Fernández T, García-López H, López Ruiz MDC, Osuna-Pérez MC. Digital and Interactive Health Interventions Minimize the Physical and Psychological Impact of Breast Cancer, Increasing Women's Quality of Life: A Systematic Review and Meta-Analysis. Cancers (Basel). 2022 Aug 26;14(17):4133. doi: 10.3390/cancers14174133. PMID: 36077670; PMCID: PMC9454975. Retrieved from: https://www.ncbi.nlm.nih.gov/pmc/articles/PMC9454975/

Oh B, Butow PN, Mullan BA, Clarke SJ, Beale PJ, Pavlakis N, Lee MS, Rosenthal DS, Larkey L, Vardy J. Effect of medical Qigong on cognitive function, quality of life, and a biomarker of inflammation in cancer patients: a randomized controlled trial. Support Care Cancer.

2012 Jun;20(6):1235-42. doi: 10.1007/s00520-011-1209-6. Epub 2011 Jun 19. PMID: 21688163.

Okajima S, Hirota A, Kimura E, Inagaki M, Tamai N, Iizaka S, Nakagami G, Mori T, Sugama J, Sanada H. Health-related quality of life and associated factors in patients with primary lymphedema. Jpn J Nurs Sci. 2013 Dec;10(2):202-11. doi: 10.1111/j.1742-7924.2012.00220.x. Epub 2012 Jul 3. PMID: 24373443. Retrieved from: https://onlinelibrary.wiley.com/doi/10.1111/j.1742-7924.2012.00220.x

Olsson Möller U, Beck I, Rydén L, Malmström M. A comprehensive approach to rehabilitation interventions following breast cancer treatment - a systematic review of systematic reviews. BMC Cancer. 2019 May 20;19(1):472. doi: 10.1186/s12885-019-5648-7. PMID: 31109309; PMCID: PMC6528312. Retrieved from: https://www.ncbi.nlm.nih.gov/pmc/articles/PMC6528312/pdf/12885_2019_Article_5648.pdf

Padmanabhan, R., Hildreth, A. J., & Laws, D. (2005). A prospective, randomized, controlled study examining binaural beat audio and pre-operative anxiety in patients undergoing general anesthesia for day case surgery. *Anesthesia, 60*(9), 874-7. Retrieved from: https://associationofanaesthetists-publications.onlinelibrary.wiley.com/doi/10.1111/j.1365-2044.2005.04287.x

Pandi-Perumal SR, Spence DW, Srivastava N, Kanchibhotla D, Kumar K, Sharma GS, Gupta R,

Batmanabane G. The Origin and Clinical Relevance of Yoga Nidra. Sleep Vigil. 2022;6(1):61-84. doi: 10.1007/s41782-022-00202-7. Epub 2022 Apr 23. PMID: 35496325; PMCID: PMC9033521. Retrieved from: https://www.ncbi.nlm.nih.gov/pmc/articles/PMC9033521/

Patel SR, Zayas J, Medina-Inojosa JR, Loprinzi C, Cathcart-Rake EJ, Bhagra A, Olson JE, Couch FJ, Ruddy KJ. Real-World Experiences With Yoga on Cancer-Related Symptoms in Women With Breast Cancer. Glob Adv Health Med. 2021 Jan 8;10:2164956120984140. doi: 10.1177/2164956120984140. PMID: 33473331; PMCID: PMC7797571. Retrieved from: https://pubmed.ncbi.nlm.nih.gov/33473331/

Pehlivan, B. , Erdoganolu, Y. , Of, N. S. , Tüzün, Ş. “The relationship between kinesiophobia, physical performance and balance in lower extremity lymphedema patients” . Türk Fizyoterapi ve Rehabilitasyon Dergisi 33 (2022): 39-47 Retrieved from: https://dergipark.org.tr/en/download/article-file/1766729

Perez CS, Mestriner C, Ribeiro LTN, Grillo FW, Lemos TW, Carneiro AA, Guirro RRJ, Guirro ECO. Relationship between lymphedema after breast cancer treatment and biophysical characteristics of the affected tissue. PLoS One. 2022 Apr 20;17(4):e0264160. doi: 10.1371/journal.pone.0264160. PMID: 35442985; PMCID: PMC9020674. Retrieved from: https://www.ncbi.nlm.nih.gov/pmc/articles/PMC9020674/

Poljsak B. Strategies for reducing or preventing the generation of oxidative stress. Oxid Med Cell Longev. 2011;2011:194586. doi: 10.1155/2011/194586. Epub 2011 Dec 10. PMID: 22191011; PMCID: PMC3236599. Retrieved from: https://www.ncbi.nlm.nih.gov/pmc/articles/PMC3236599/

Program Significantly Impacts Women With Breast Cancer-Related Lymphedema, Study Says. (2010, Jan. 4). Retrieved from: https://rehabpub.com/industry-news/research/program-significantly-impacts-women-with-breast-cancer-related-lymphedema-study-says/

Qigong. (29 July 2022). Retrieved from: https://www.mskcc.org/cancer-care/integrative-medicine/therapies/qigong

Raghuraj P, Telles S. Immediate effect of specific nostril manipulating yoga breathing practices on autonomic and respiratory variables. Appl Psychophysiol Biofeedback. 2008 Jun;33(2):65-75. doi: 10.1007/s10484-008-9055-0. Epub 2008 Mar 18. PMID: 18347974. Retrieved from: https://www.researchgate.net/profile/Raghuraj-Puthige/publication/5504433_Immediate_Effect_of_Specific_Nostril_Manipulating_Yoga_Breathing_Practices_on_Autonomic_and_Respiratory_Variables/links/60f90eec169a1a0103ab3c1d/Immediate-Effect-of-Specific-Nostril-Manipulating-Yoga-Breathing-Practices-on-Autonomic-and-Respiratory-Variables.pdf

Redwine, L. S., Henry, B. L., Pung, M. A., Wilson, K., Chinh, K., Knight, B., Jain, S., Rutledge, T., Greenberg, B., Maisel, A., & Mills, P. J. (2016). Pilot Randomized Study of a Gratitude Journaling Intervention on Heart Rate Variability and Inflammatory Biomarkers in Patients With Stage B Heart Failure. *Psychosomatic medicine*, *78*(6), 667–676. https://doi.org/10.1097/PSY.0000000000000316 Retrieved from: https://www.ncbi.nlm.nih.gov/pmc/articles/PMC4927423/

Reich RR, Lengacher CA, Klein TW, Newton C, Shivers S, Ramesar S, Alinat CB, Paterson C, Le A, Park JY, Johnson-Mallard V, Elias M, Moscoso M, Goodman M, Kip KE. A Randomized Controlled Trial of the Effects of Mindfulness-Based Stress Reduction (MBSR[BC]) on Levels of Inflammatory Biomarkers Among Recovering Breast Cancer Survivors. Biol Res Nurs. 2017 Jul;19(4):456-464. doi: 10.1177/1099800417707268. Epub 2017 May 1. PMID: 28460534; PMCID: PMC5942506. Retrieved from: https://www.ncbi.nlm.nih.gov/pmc/articles/PMC5942506/

Ridner SH. The psycho-social impact of lymphedema. Lymphat Res Biol. 2009;7(2):109-12. doi: 10.1089/lrb.2009.0004. PMID: 19534633; PMCID: PMC2904185. Retrieved from: https://www.ncbi.nlm.nih.gov/pmc/articles/PMC2904185/

Rio-Alamos C, Montefusco-Siegmund R, Cañete T, Sotomayor J, Fernandez-Teruel A. Acute Relaxation Response Induced by Tibetan Singing Bowl Sounds:

A Randomized Controlled Trial. Eur J Investig Health Psychol Educ. 2023 Jan 29;13(2):317-330. doi: 10.3390/ejihpe13020024. PMID: 36826208; PMCID: PMC9955072. https://www.ncbi.nlm.nih.gov/pmc/articles/PMC9955072/

Río-González Á, Molina-Rueda F, Palacios-Ceña D, Alguacil-Diego IM. Comparing the experience of individuals with primary and secondary lymphoedema: A qualitative study. Braz J Phys Ther. 2021 Mar-Apr;25(2):203-213. doi: 10.1016/j.bjpt.2020.05.009. Epub 2020 Jun 1. PMID: 32518025; PMCID: PMC7990727. Retrieved from: https://www.ncbi.nlm.nih.gov/pmc/articles/PMC7990727/

Risk and Protective Factors (n.d.). Retrieved from: https://www.cdc.gov/violenceprevention/childabuseandneglect/riskprotectivefactors.html

Russo MA, Santarelli DM, O'Rourke D. The physiological effects of slow breathing in the healthy human. Breathe (Sheff). 2017 Dec;13(4):298-309. doi: 10.1183/20734735.009817. PMID: 29209423; PMCID: PMC5709795. Retrieved from: https://www.ncbi.nlm.nih.gov/pmc/articles/PMC5709795/

Rustad JK, David D, Currier MB. Cancer and post-traumatic stress disorder: diagnosis, pathogenesis and treatment considerations. Palliat Support Care. 2012 Sep;10(3):213-23. doi: 10.1017/S1478951511000897. Epub 2012 Mar 22. PMID: 22436138.

Ryan, T. (2019). The Nature of care in the management of Lymphoedema; not without laughter! *Journal of Lymphoedema,* 14(1), 54–55. Retrieved from: https://lymphoedemaeducation.com.au/wp-content/uploads/2019/08/11.-The-nature-of-care-in-the-management-of-lymphoedema-not-without-laughter.pdf

Sahbaz Pirincci C, Cihan E, Borman P, Dalyan M. Does Fear of Movement Affect Fatigue and Quality of Life in Lower Extremity Lymphedema? Lymphat Res Biol. 2022 Dec 29. doi: 10.1089/lrb.2022.0050. Epub ahead of print. PMID: 36580543. Retrieved from: https://pubmed.ncbi.nlm.nih.gov/36580543/

Saraswathi V, Latha S, Niraimathi K, Vidhubala E. Managing Lymphedema, Increasing Range of Motion, and Quality of Life through Yoga Therapy among Breast Cancer Survivors: A Systematic Review. Int J Yoga. 2021 Jan-Apr;14(1):3-17. doi: 10.4103/ijoy.IJOY_73_19. Epub 2021 Feb 5. PMID: 33840972; PMCID: PMC8023442. Retrieved from: https://www.ncbi.nlm.nih.gov/pmc/articles/PMC8023442/

Segerstrom SC, Miller GE. Psychological stress and the human immune system: a meta-analytic study of 30 years of inquiry. Psychol Bull. 2004 Jul;130(4):601-30. doi: 10.1037/0033-2909.130.4.601. PMID: 15250815; PMCID: PMC1361287. Retrieved from: https://www.researchgate.net/profile/Suzanne-Segerstrom/publication/247293833_Psychological_stress_and_the_immune_system_a_meta-analytic_study_of_30_ years_of_inquiry/links/00b495201270d4dd72000000/Psychological-stress-and-the-immune-system-a-meta-analytic-study-of-30-years-of-inquiry.pdf

Shani P, Walter E. Acceptability and Use of Mind-Body Interventions Among African American Cancer Survivors: An Integrative Review. Integr Cancer Ther. 2022 Jan-Dec;21:15347354221103275. doi: 10.1177/15347354221103275. PMID: 35786041; PMCID: PMC9251965. Retrieved from: https://www.ncbi.nlm.nih.gov/pmc/articles/PMC9251965/

Shim, J., Yeun, Y., Kim, H., & Kim, S. (2017). Effects of manual lymph drainage for abdomen on the brain activity of subjects with psychological stress. *Journal of Physical Therapy Science, 29*, 491 - 494. Retrieved from: https://pdfs.semanticscholar.org/fe95/4e425cd9a9c6835de4eddf398953188345d2.pdf?gl=1*5sx33s*ga*MTE0MjEzMzA3NS4xNjc2MjM3NzU4*ga H7P4ZT52H5*MTY3OTQ1OTM3NC41LjEuMTY3OTQ2MTA2OS4wLjAuMA..

Siems WG, Brenke R, Beier A, Grune T. Oxidative stress in chronic lymphoedema. QJM. 2002 Dec;95(12):803-9. doi: 10.1093/qjmed/95.12.803. PMID: 12454323. https://pubmed.ncbi.nlm.nih.gov/12454323/

Singh MV, Chapleau MW, Harwani SC, Abboud FM. The immune system and hypertension. Immunol Res. 2014 Aug;59(1-3):243-53. doi: 10.1007/s12026-014-8548-

6. PMID: 24847766; PMCID: PMC4313884. Retrieved from: https://www.ncbi.nlm.nih.gov/pmc/articles/PMC4313884/

Smith, S. (2018). *5-4-3-2-1 coping technique for anxiety.* Retrieved from: https://www.urmc.rochester.edu/behavioral-health-partners/bhp-blog/april-2018/5-4-3-2-1-coping-technique-for-anxiety.aspx

Snyder M, Tseng Y, Brandt C, Croghan C, Hanson S, Constantine R, Kirby L. A glider swing intervention for people with dementia. Geriatr Nurs. 2001 Mar-Apr;22(2):86-90. doi: 10.1067/mgn.2001.115197. PMID: 11326215.

Sohl SJ, Dietrich MS, Wallston KA, Ridner SH. A randomized controlled trial of expressive writing in breast cancer survivors with lymphedema. Psychol Health. 2017 Jul;32(7):826-842. doi: 10.1080/08870446.2017.1307372. Epub 2017 Mar 30. Erratum in: Psychol Health. 2017 Sep;32(9):1167. PMID: 28355890; PMCID: PMC5571730. Retrieved from:

https://www.tandfonline.com/doi/full/10.1080/08870446.2017.1307372?scroll=top&needAccess=true

Spada GE, Masiero M, Pizzoli SFM, Pravettoni G. Heart Rate Variability Biofeedback in Cancer Patients: A Scoping Review. Behav Sci (Basel). 2022 Oct 11;12(10):389. doi: 10.3390/bs12100389. PMID: 36285958; PMCID: PMC9598295. Retrieved from: https://www.ncbi.nlm.nih.gov/pmc/articles/PMC9598295/

Speck RM, Gross CR, Hormes JM, Ahmed RL, Lytle LA, Hwang WT, Schmitz KH. Changes in the Body Image and Relationship Scale following a one-year strength training trial for breast cancer survivors with or at risk for lymphedema. Breast Cancer Res Treat. 2010 Jun;121(2):421-30. doi: 10.1007/s10549-009-0550-7. Epub 2009 Sep 22. PMID: 19771507. Retrieved from: https://paulogentil.com/pdf/Changes%20in%20the%20Body%20Image%20and%20Relationship%20Scale%20following%20a%20one-year%20strength%20training%20trial%20for%20breast%20cancer%2-0survivors%20with%20or%20at%20risk%20for%20lymphedema.pdf

Stephens MA, Wand G. Stress and the HPA axis: role of glucocorticoids in alcohol dependence. Alcohol Res. 2012;34(4):468-83. PMID: 23584113; PMCID: PMC3860380.

Retrieved from: https://www.ncbi.nlm.nih.gov/pmc/articles/PMC3860380

Tamam N, Al-Mugren KS, Alrebdi HI, Sulieman A, Abdelbasset WK. Evaluating the Quality of Life and Sleep Quality in Saudi Women with Breast Cancer-Related Lymphedema: A Cross-Sectional Correlational Study. Integr Cancer Ther. 2021 Jan-Dec;20:15347354211046192. doi: 10.1177/15347354211046192. PMID: 34541909; PMCID: PMC8450611. Retrieved from: https://www.ncbi.nlm.nih.gov/pmc/articles/PMC8450611/

Tanzmeister S, Rominger C, Weber B, Tatschl JM, Schwerdtfeger AR. Singing at 0.1 Hz as a Resonance Frequency Intervention to Reduce Cardiovascular Stress Reactivity? Front Psychiatry. 2022 Apr 27;13:876344. doi: 10.3389/fpsyt.2022.876344. PMID: 35573368; PMCID: PMC9091602. Retrieved from: https://www.ncbi.nlm.nih.gov/pmc/articles/PMC9091602/

Telles S, Vishwakarma B, Gupta RK, Balkrishna A. Changes in Shape and Size Discrimination and State Anxiety After Alternate-Nostril Yoga Breathing and Breath Awareness in One Session Each. Med Sci Monit Basic Res. 2019 Apr 22;25:121-127. doi: 10.12659/MSMBR.914956. PMID: 31006767; PMCID: PMC6496972. Retrieved from: https://www.ncbi.nlm.nih.gov/pmc/articles/PMC6496972/

Thomas R, Gifford W, Hammond C. Writing toward well-being: A qualitative study of community-based workshops with breast cancer survivors. Can Oncol Nurs J. 2017 May 1;27(2):178-185. doi: 10.5737/23688076272178185. PMID: 31148636; PMCID: PMC6516224. Retrieved from: https://www.ncbi.nlm.nih.gov/pmc/articles/PMC6516224/pdf/conj-27-2-178.pdf

Toole A. & Craighead L. (2016). Brief self-compassion meditation training for body image distress in young adult women. Body Image. 19. 104-112. 10.1016/j.bodyim.2016.09.001. Retrieved from https:/self-compassion.org/wp-content/uploads/2017/01/Toole2016.pdf

Trivedi GY, Patel V, Shah MH, Dhok MJ, Bhoyania K. Comparative study of the impact of active meditation protocol and silence meditation on heart rate variability and mood in women. Int J Yoga 2020;13:255-60. Retrieved from: https://www.ncbi.nlm.nih.gov/pmc/articles/PMC7735506/pdf/IJY-13-255.pdf

Trivedi, G. Y., & Saboo, B. (2021). Bhramari Pranayama - A simple lifestyle intervention to reduce heart rate, enhance the lung function and immunity. *Journal of Ayurveda and integrative medicine*, *12*(3), 562–564. https://doi.org/10.1016/j.jaim.2021.07.004

Twal WO, Wahlquist AE, Balasubramanian S. Yogic breathing when compared to attention control reduces the levels of pro-inflammatory biomarkers in saliva: a pilot randomized controlled trial. BMC Complement Altern Med. 2016 Aug 18;16:294. doi: 10.1186/s12906-016-1286-7. PMID: 27538513; PMCID: PMC4991069. Retrieved from: https://www.ncbi.nlm.nih.gov/pmc/articles/PMC4991069/

Twohig-Bennett C, Jones A. The health benefits of the great outdoors: A systematic review and meta-analysis of greenspace exposure and health outcomes. Environ Res. 2018 Oct;166:628-637. doi: 10.1016/j.envres.2018.06.030. Epub 2018 Jul 5. PMID: 29982151; PMCID: PMC6562165. Retrieved from: https://www.ncbi.nlm.nih.gov/pmc/articles/PMC6562165/

Vago DR, Silbersweig DA. Self-awareness, self-regulation, and self-transcendence (S-ART): a framework for understanding the neurobiological mechanisms of mindfulness. Front Hum Neurosci. 2012 Oct 25;6:296. doi: 10.3389/fnhum.2012.00296. PMID: 23112770; PMCID: PMC3480633. Retrieved from: https://www.ncbi.nlm.nih.gov/pmc/articles/PMC3480633/

Valois BA, Young TE, Melsome E. Assessing the feasibility of using acupuncture and moxibustion to improve quality of life for cancer survivors with upper body lymphoedema. Eur J Oncol Nurs 2012;16:301-309. 22.

Vaschillo, E. G., Vaschillo, B., Pandina, R. J., and Bates, M. E. (2011). Resonances in the cardiovascular system caused by rhythmical muscle tension. *Psychophysiology* 48, 927–936. doi: 10.1111/j.1469-8986.2010.01156.x Retrieved from: https://www.ncbi.nlm.nih.gov/pmc/articles/PMC3094735/

Vinson, J., Powers, J., & Mosesso K. Weighted blankets: Anxiety reduction in adult patients receiving chemotherapy. *Clin J Oncology Nursing, 24*(4), 360-368. Retrieved from: https://pubmed.ncbi.nlm.nih.gov/32678376/

Wang C, Yang M, Fan Y, Pei X. Moxibustion as a Therapy for Breast Cancer-Related Lymphedema in Female Adults: A Preliminary Randomized Controlled Trial. Integr Cancer Ther. 2019 Jan-Dec;18:1534735419866919. doi:

10.1177/1534735419866919. PMID: 31422715; PMCID: PMC6700867. Retrieved from: https://www.ncbi.nlm.nih.gov/pmc/articles/PMC6700867/

Weitzberg E, Lundberg JO. Humming greatly increases nasal nitric oxide. Am J Respir Crit Care Med. 2002 Jul 15;166(2):144-5. doi: 10.1164/rccm.200202-138BC. PMID: 12119224. Retrieved from: https://www.atsjournals.org/doi/full/10.1164/rccm.200202-138BC

Wen, Y., Yan, Q., Pan, Y. et al. Medical empirical research on forest bathing (*Shinrin-yoku*): a systematic review. *Environ Health Prev Med* 24, 70 (2019). https://doi.org/10.1186/s12199-019-0822-8 Retrieved from: https://environhealthprevmed.biomedcentral.com/articles/10.1186/s12199-019-0822-8

Wilkinson SM, Love SB, Westcombe AM, Gambles MA, Burgess CC, Cargill A, Young T, Maher EJ, Ramirez AJ. Effectiveness of aromatherapy massage in the management of anxiety and depression in patients with cancer: a multicenter randomized controlled trial. J Clin Oncol. 2007 Feb 10;25(5):532-9. doi: 10.1200/JCO.2006.08.9987. PMID: 17290062. Retrieved from: https://ascopubs.org/doi/10.1200/JCO.2006.08.9987?url_ver=Z39.88-2003&rfr_id=ori:rid:crossref.org&rfr_dat=cr_pub%20%200pubmed

Wilson JM, Haliwa I, Lee J, Shook NJ. The role of dispositional mindfulness in the fear-avoidance model of pain. PLoS One. 2023 Jan 27;18(1):e0280740. doi: 10.1371/journal.pone.0280740. PMID: 36706069; PMCID: PMC9882899. Retrieved from: https://www.ncbi.nlm.nih.gov/pmc/articles/PMC9882899/pdf/pone.0280740.pdf

Wood, J. V., Perunovic, W. Q., & Lee, J. W. (2009). Positive self-statements: Power for some, peril for others. *Psychology Science, 20*(7), 860-6. Retrieved from: https://www.uni-muenster.de/imperia/md/content/psyifp/aeechterhoff/wintersemester2011-12/seminarthemenfelderdersozialpsychologie/04_wood_etal_selfstatements_psychscience2009.pdf

Yang JC, Huang LH, Wu SC, Kuo PJ, Wu YC, Wu CJ, Lin CW, Tsai PY, Hsieh CH. Lymphaticovenous Anastomosis Supermicrosurgery Decreases Oxidative Stress and Increases Antioxidant Capacity in the Serum of Lymphedema Patients. J Clin Med. 2021 Apr 6;10(7):1540. doi: 10.3390/jcm10071540. PMID: 33917571; PMCID: PMC8038828. Retrieved from: https://www.ncbi.nlm.nih.gov/pmc/articles/PMC8038828/

Yuan Y, Arcucci V, Levy SM, Achen MG. Modulation of Immunity by Lymphatic Dysfunction in Lymphedema. Front Immunol. 2019 Jan 29;10:76. doi: 10.3389/fimmu.2019.00076. PMID: 30761143; PMCID: PMC6361763. Retrieved from: https://www.ncbi.nlm.nih.gov/pmc/articles/PMC6361763/

Zahourek RP. Commentary on "Exploring the effects of walking the labyrinth". J Holist Nurs. 2006 Jun;24(2):111-2. doi: 10.1177/0898010106287561. PMID: 16740900.

Zampi, D. D. (2016). Efficacy of theta binaural beats for the treatment of chronic pain. *Altern Ther Health Medicine, 22*(1), 32-8.

Zhao, W., Li, H., Zhu, X., & Ge, T. (2020). Effect of birdsong soundscape on perceived restorativeness in an Urban Park. *Int J Environ Res Public Health, 17*(16), 5659. Retrieved from: https://www.ncbi.nlm.nih.gov/pmc/articles/PMC7459586/

Zou L, Sasaki JE, Wei GX, Huang T, Yeung AS, Neto OB, Chen KW, Hui SS. Effects of Mind-Body Exercises (Tai Chi/Yoga) on Heart Rate Variability Parameters and Perceived Stress: A Systematic Review with Meta-Analysis of Randomized Controlled Trials. J Clin Med. 2018 Oct 31;7(11):404. doi: 10.3390/jcm7110404. PMID: 30384420; PMCID: PMC6262541. Retrieved from: https://www.ncbi.nlm.nih.gov/pmc/articles/PMC6262541/

Made in the USA
Coppell, TX
26 July 2023

19598532R00125